Human Services in the Network So

The Internet and the many applications it supports continue to transform and expand the ways in which it is possible to relate, communicate, collaborate, and perform human service work. In this book, human service researchers and practitioners explore major opportunities and challenges to well being, social justice, and human service work that technology use in everyday life has exposed. Drawing on the latest research their contributions examine issues associated with human service practices in the network society, including: the implications of an expanded capacity to share human service data across agency and national boundaries; ethical issues associated with the use of remote sensing and surveillance technologies (e.g. the satellite tracking of offenders, and telecare services for older people); the risks and benefits of social network sites including issues associated with online privacy, intimacy, and safety; and the influence of technology-mediated services on human relationships and the sense of 'being present' with another person.

Human Services in the Network Society will be of considerable interest to human service professionals, academics and researchers who are concerned about the social impact of networked technologies.

This book was previously published as a special issue of the *Journal of Technology in Human Services*.

Neil Ballantyne is a New Zealand based Independent Researcher and Consultant and visiting Senior Research Fellow at the School of Applied Social Sciences, University of Strathclyde, UK.

Walter LaMendola is a Professor and Chair of the Doctoral Program at the Graduate School of Social Work, University of Denver, USA.

Human Services in the Network Society

Edited by
Neil Ballantyne and Walter LaMendola

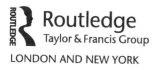

Routledge
Taylor & Francis Group

LONDON AND NEW YORK

First published 2012 by Routledge

2 Park Square, Milton Park, Abingdon, Oxfordshire OX14 4RN
711 Third Avenue, New York, NY 10017

Routledge is an imprint of the Taylor & Francis Group, an informa business

First issued in paperback 2018

British Library Cataloguing in Publication Data
A catalogue record for this book is available from the British Library

ISBN13: 978-0-415-69009-6 (hbk)
ISBN13: 978-1-138-38312-8 (pbk)

Typeset in Garamond
by Taylor & Francis Books

Disclaimer
The publisher would like to make readers aware that the chapters in this book are referred to as articles as they had been in the special issue. The publisher accepts responsibility for any inconsistencies that may have arisen in the course of preparing this volume for print.

Contents

Introduction: Human Services
in the Network Society

NEIL BALLANTYNE AND WALTER LAMENDOLA

At the turn of the century, Manuel Castells – the preeminent sociologist of the Internet – argued that, in order to understand the changes associated with the information age that were rapidly diffusing throughout society, a new sociology was required. A sociology based on empirical observation, rigorous theorizing and clear communication about the nature of the emerging network society (Castells, 2010). This new understanding was needed, argued Castells (2000, p693) *"...because without understanding, people, rightly, will block change, and we may lose the extraordinary potential of creativity embedded into the values and technologies of the Information Age."*

The chapters that follow are all directly connected to or influenced by an international research symposium held in Glasgow, Scotland, in September 2009. The symposium was hosted by the Institute for Advanced Studies and organized by *Connected Practice*: a research unit within the Glasgow School of Social Work. The symposium was titled "Human Services in the Network Society," and its purpose was to provide a focus for an international exchange about the changes, challenges, and opportunities that networked technologies are bringing to the lives of the users of human services and to the practice of human service practitioners. What was innovative about the symposium was not that it brought together human services academics, managers and workers to talk about the implications of information and communications technologies (ICTs), because HUSITA (http://www.husita.org/) and other organizations have been hosting conferences on human services and ICTs for many years. What was new was the explicit focus on *networked technologies* and the exploration of the emergence of what has been termed the *network society* for the practice of human service practitioners.

Walter LaMendola (1988) was among the first human service practitioners to document human service activity in what we now call the network society. In 1985 he identified over 300 separate electronic network sites in Denver, Colorado, alone. He classified human service activity in networks at that time into six categories: public service networks, community networks, human service organization networks, professional networks, and client centered networks (p. 240). He concluded by saying that the idea that groups of people can form voluntary communities circumscribed by areas of intellectual, emotional, social, sexual, or political interest is both compelling and real to those who use electronic networks. For the most part, in electronic networking the transformative powers of the technology are usually more vivid and clear than in other implementations of information technology (p. 242).

The concept of the network society as first described by Van Dijk (1991) and elaborated in detail over three volumes by Castells (2000a, 2000b, 2004) argues that the use of electronic networks are fundamentally altering the nature of societies, cultures, and economies in the developed world. They are transforming the ways in which it is possible for humans to relate, communicate, collaborate, conduct trade, and work. In the context of the human services, electronic network use is transforming the ways in which we organize and deliver human services. In fact, they are altering and generating new forms of social life. In turn, this is opening up new channels for expressing social solidarity and, at the same time, opening new opportunities for social disorder.

In the 1990s, when the Internet began to emerge as a significant societal phenomenon, the media and the public became fascinated by its promise to transform society for good or ill. Academic commentators also began to sketch both utopian and dystopian visions of the future of the network society. The utopians described brave new worlds where technology ushered in a new electronic democracy: sweeping aside the traditional boundaries and inequities of sex, class, and race; and empowering individuals to access information and engage in online communities with other *netizens* from anywhere in the world. Meanwhile, those with a more skeptical view warned of social isolation; the further fragmentation of family and community; and the erosion of privacy, as government, business and criminal interests surveilled and monitored citizen behavior on the net.

Although today we can point to examples in support of both of these views, overall, the empirical evidence suggests that neither was entirely accurate. As Benkler (2006, p357) argues, *"while neither view had it completely right, it was the dystopian view that got it especially wrong"*. Networked communications and social media are influencing family, community and social life but in complex and subtle ways. For many years the work of Wellman and colleagues associated with Netlab at the University of Toronto, along with the more recent studies conducted as part of the Pew Internet and American Life project, have made a significant contribution to a deeper understanding of how technology is mediating new forms of emerging networked sociality. Wellman (2001) named this pattern "networked individualism."

According to Wellman, rather than the collapse of community, Internet mediated communications are contributing to the creation of new forms of community of choice, based on personal networks. What is shifting is the reliance on densely knit, tightly bound, traditional communities of place and their replacement (at least for those in developed economies) with personal communities of strong and loose ties. The new forms of community are managed and maintained by a combination of offline face-to-face encounters and online network technologies. Examples of the technologies people use continues to expand and now includes mobile telephony, text messaging, social network sites, e-mail, and instant messaging.

But what are the implications of these changes for the organization and delivery of human services? How can the affordances of networked technology be harnessed for the delivery of human services? And, what are the emerging risks and benefits for human services in the Network Society? In the remainder of this chapter we will touch on just a few of the themes and issues associated with these questions, and at the same time introduce the chapters that follow which will explore a few of the questions in greater depth.

NETWORKED INFORMATION

Networked information is an umbrella term referring to the prolific expansion of possible human relationships and actionable knowledge available through participation in Internet and mobile communication services. There has been a steady, well-documented growth of visible networked information; and, at the same time, the growth of undocumented hidden networked information, for example, the hidden web is substantial and has been estimated in size to equal more than 500 times the visible web (Barbosa, 2010). Networked information can take many forms, from one-to-one communications, such as those that dominate most e-mail, to one-to-many communications, such as is typical in social media. Mobile devices and their applications have experienced the same two types of network information development.

Visible uses of network information are dominated by individual communications and searches, mostly through static forms such as websites. Invisible uses include corporate commercial uses as well as protected health and human service information. The hidden web also supports public agency activities and clandestine surveillance. LaMendola, Ballantyne, and Daly (2010) explored practitioner use of networked services in local authorities to build ties among practitioners and increase access to repositories of evidence-based practice. Their experience exposed a number of issues with facilitating individualized network access within institutions located in the hidden human service web.

Mainly, human service organizations are relatively closed systems that are struggling to learn how, and in what manner, they might harness the more open architecture of networked communications. In this volume, Schoech highlights the critical nature of this problem by addressing inter-operability issues intersecting the invisible human service web that – unless dealt with rather immediately – will continue to limit institutional service development; sharing of health and human service information; and, by fiat, the ability of institutional human services to create knowledge based on practitioner wisdom. Schoech argues that like other businesses, there is a growing need for human service agencies to share data across organizational, state, and national boundaries and to increase the extent of interoperability between systems.

Networked technologies have been at the heart of the transformational potential of many 20th century technological innovations including railroads, highways, telephony, and the Internet. In each case the gradual emergence of standards to support effective interoperability, or service integration across the network, has been fundamental. Schoech's article explores the potential for an interoperable, global human service delivery infrastructure and draws on exemplars from business to explore three possible models for human services interoperability: a loosely linked networked model (based on Web 2.0, cloud computing, and iPhone apps); a network model (based on the highly integrated, real-time information exchange used by industries such as the travel industry); and a top–down model (based on the data-protection concerns of industries like the banking industry). Whether or not human services adopt one or a blend of these models will have far-reaching consequences for the way in which services are delivered, and for the operational ethos of human service organizations.

Although Schoech focuses on information and knowledge sharing within and between human service organizations, networked technologies are also being used by citizens and users of human services to forge their own social support networks, to share information and knowledge, and sometimes to challenge the former monopoly on expertise claimed by human service organizations. Indeed, the first decades of networked information development focused largely on traditions of sharing explicit and codified knowledge, such as libraries or support groups might do. However, the emerging value of networks is now recognized to be their use of sharing tacit knowledge, and of empowering ordinary people through social media. Social media is also being used by not-for-profit organizations to enhance public awareness of social causes and raise funds (e.g. http://summerofsocialgood.com/ and http://www.charitywater.org/). Research has uncovered the ways in which networked technologies can be harnessed in response to natural disasters, such as in Haiti, where US government agencies employed wikis and collaborative social media as the main knowledge discovery and management tools (Yates & Paquette, 2011). And social media has also been used to assist homeless persons find food and shelter (Cary, 2011).

NETWORKED SERVICE DELIVERY

The focus in human services has grown from dealing with the ways in which electronic networks are influencing and might continue to influence the structure and exchange of information to the impact of networked technologies on forms of service delivery. Human service delivery has encountered the enormous expansion of objects in the social world and the mobility that accompanies it. In many developed countries, service access and utilization is based on the use of cars, smart phones, texting, and Internet services. People leave trails of personal and everyday data behind them without notice. The data is accumulated and aggregated and becomes part of databases which parallel human service databases. People use databases freely themselves, like Twitter or Facebook, not only to portray reactions, experiences, and accomplishments, but also to engage in social support. In such an environment, much of what now constitutes the human service delivery system must respond and facilitate, not direct or command, as meaning is constructed by individual participation in the network and by individualized networking activities. Changes in forms of service delivery are underway.

So far, many human services begin engaging in network services by modeling programs in the format in which they already exist. Internet based services have proliferated for governmental human services, behavioral health services, and services provided by community based organizations. Webb, Joseph, Yardley, and Michie (2010) reviewed web-based behavioral health interventions that sought to affect specific behavioral changes. One of the three major characteristics that contributed to higher effect sizes was "mode of delivery". However, their coding of this area was constrained by the fact that the mode of delivery was usually not specified clearly. Still, in all cases, the service was networked.

Indeed, most human services in developed countries now also exist in a networked format. Human services are rushing to use forms of social media (Chou, Hunt, Beckjord, Moser, & Hesse, 2009; LaMendola, 2011), gaming (Wilkinson, Ang, & Goh, 2008), and on-line communities (Enos, 2008). Currently, systems are being developed that use the network to assess status and motivation; monitor recovery progress; provide access to self-help meetings, and manage tasks relating to self assessments and goals (VanDeMark, Burrell, LaMendola et al., 2010; Cucciare, Weingardt, & Humphreys, 2009). Studies so far have found significant positive change in areas of mental health assessment, prevention, and treatment (Cuijpers, Donker, van Straten, & Andersson,

2010; Newman, Koif, Przeworski, & Llera, 2010). This is particularly true if the service is supported by a human service worker (Newman, Szkodny, Llera, & Przeworski, 2011).

Included in this volume are three chapters dealing with networked service delivery. One offers a critique of networked services that may diminish relational aspects of the human service while two others offer insights into contrasting but technologically sophisticated domains of human service delivery that have been under-investigated: (a) the electronic monitoring of offenders and (b) telecare services for people with health or disability issues. In each of these domains human service practitioners have come to rely on remote monitoring, sensing, and surveillance: in one case, for the purposes of technologically delivered care; and in the other for the purposes of offender management, community safety, and control.

Nellis describes emerging patterns in the satellite tracking of offenders using systems that go beyond the retrospective monitoring of offenders movements to systems that can track their precise location in "real time." He directly addresses the ethical implications and changed relationship between supervisors and supervised in this technology-mediated practice. Nellis inexorably draws our attention to the connections between the network society and the surveillance society. While he recognizes the value of a technology that aims to support community safety at the same time as it keeps offenders out of institutions, he also argues that this technology fundamentally alters the relational aspects of probation work with offenders. While there are certainly social benefits to surveillance, Nellis may agree with McCluskey (2005) that in this case "to be reduced to a moving dot on a screen-map, to be watched as a mere simulation is not, as a therapist might put it, 'to be met as a person.'"

As remote sensing technology has developed for monitoring offenders, parallel systems have also developed in the field of telemedicine and telecare. Telecare services offer the prospect of a technology that enables people with health or disability issues (older people in particular) to remain in their own home supported by remote sensing and communication technologies that alert caregivers to problems or issues. This book includes two chapters exploring telecare in the Scottish context. Andrew Eccles adopts a critical stance, questioning government rationale for a policy commitment to telecare driven, he argues, by fiscal imperatives to contain service costs and improve service delivery efficiencies. In particular he highlights the potential of telecare to reduce fiscal costs by replacing institutional care. At the same time, he notes the increase in human relational costs by reducing human contact and isolating recipients within their own homes. He also urges human service managers and practitioners to reflect on telecare practice using ethical frameworks that are congruent with an "ethic of care" and the relational aspects of human service provision. Ethical issues in the implementation of telecare, he argues, must be considered in their rich, complex, human, and relational context.

In the second chapter on telecare, Beale and colleagues report on an empirical evaluation of the Scottish Government telecare development program. Their findings are broadly supportive of the program, estimating that 1,200 hospital admissions and over 500 delayed discharges from hospital were avoided. Data from the recipients of the service indicated that all felt safer as a result of the program, two thirds felt more independent, and very few felt lonelier. In addition, the informal caregivers of program recipients were very positive about the program and felt reassured by it. They conclude that, their findings, like the findings of prior research, support the view that telecare can "lead to improvements in patients' perceptions of the quality of care they receive and ultimately their quality of life." Although this empirical data might seem to provide reassurance on the ethical issues raised by Eccles, the authors are careful to point to the limitations of their research design, and the need to continue to collect data and monitor and evaluate telecare programs if we are to maximize benefits and minimize risks.

RISKS AND BENEFITS OF THE NETWORK SOCIETY

Arguably all technical innovations – from the steam engine, to television, to the Internet – are associated with new social benefits, and new social risks. Industrialization brought sweeping societal changes including urbanization, overcrowding, pollution and the most rapid growth in standards of living in human history. The television enabled mass communication, bringing news of world events into the living rooms of ordinary people. Yet at the same time, it was implicated in the fragmentation of community, and steep falls in civic engagement (Putnam, 2000). Now, the Internet is ushering in an information age where individuals using networked technologies can find almost instant answers to almost any questions from the comfort of their home; or, using Internet connected mobile devices, from anywhere within reach of a wireless network. Human service workers connect electronically with colleagues and clients and exchange information and ideas at a distance. Citizens use social media to maintain intimate relations with family and friends, sharing the minutiae of daily life on social network sites like Facebook or microblogging systems like Twitter. At the same time, this new networked public sphere is generating new tensions, such as, reconfiguring the relationship between the private sphere and the networked public sphere; opening up new risks from networked commercial and criminal organizations; and new legislative and ethical debates on the relationship between citizens and government.

In a classic study of the social history of the telephone in American society the sociologist Claude Fischer (1992) studied the social outcomes of this, now taken for granted, technology. Early commentators on the likely social impact of the telephone put forward dystopian predictions that it would lead to the end of local community, or negatively influence the psychology of telephone users (the constant possibility of unannounced telephone calls making them tense, alert and edgy). These views were rivaled by utopian visions of a new telephonic 'brotherhood of man' made possible by a technology that enabled intimate person-to-person voice communication between individuals located anywhere in the world. Fischer's study concluded that as telephone users came to adopt and adapt this innovative new communications medium, it was successfully accommodated into social life, both shaped by and in turn shaping social practices. In other words, Americans simply used the affordances of this new communication device to pursue pre-existing social ends (mainly to maintain contact with existing family and friends) with greater vigour. We cannot conclude that the outcomes for the Internet and social media will be as benign, although the emerging data is surprisingly similar in nature. Fischer's main point is that the wave of technology is not a tsunami that overwhelms human society, but a force that can be channeled and shaped by human agency.

For example, a Pew Internet and American Life survey on the influence of technology on family life found a majority of American adults agreeing that technology permits their families to be as close, or closer, than their families were when they grew up (Kennedy et al., 2008). Most stated the Internet had not altered the amount of time spent with friends and family, and the majority was satisfied with family life. There was evidence that Internet time seemed more likely to be taken from time spent watching television (especially for young adults), and that for some, family time was prioritized at the expense of time on hobbies or clubs. However, the impact of the Internet on blurring the boundaries between home and work was evident, as one in five of those employed said the internet had increased the amount of time that they spent working from home, and one in ten that it had increased the amount of time they spent working from the office.

Contemporary struggles between different interest groups (governmental, industrial, and civil rights) about Internet privacy; online child protection; data-sharing; intellectual property, and surveillance, all attest to a lively debate amongst citizens and other stakeholders in the network society. The issues being debated may be prompted by new social practices made possible by technology, but the values underlying the debates are familiar, in that they are about the balance of power between citizens and the state, i.e., privacy; freedom of expression; protection from unnecessary surveillance; and human rights. At the time of writing, the United Nations has entered the debate by arguing that access to the Internet is a fundamental human right enabling freedom of expression and communication and a range of other human rights (United Nations, 2011).

Social network sites (e.g. MySpace and Facebook) have become a major locus for the development and maintenance of online relationships and information exchange between family members, friends, and acquaintances. At the time of writing, membership of Facebook stands at around 600 million users. To put that figure into perspective, the total number of Internet users in the world in 2002 was less than the current membership of Facebook. Social network sites have also become a major focus for researchers trying to unravel the impact of the new media on interpersonal communications and exchanges. Many of the issues surrounding the use of these sites are familiar to psychologists. They are issues of interpersonal relationships, such as, trust, intimacy, privacy, identity, and self-presentation. However, the nature of networked public space gives these face-to-face interpersonal dilemmas a new twist, and users sometimes fall foul of the unexpected features of the online interface. Our final three chapters are concerned with the risks and the benefits of the network society for individual, family, and social life and selected implications of those risks and benefits for human service practitioners.

In their chapter, Houghton and Joinson report on findings of a study to explore Facebook users' perceptions of friendship and privacy in the social network site. They identify the problems of managing the boundaries around information sharing that users need to learn to be effective users of online spaces now and in the future. Still on the theme of social network sites, Ballantyne, Duncalf, and Daly discuss the use of these sites by children and young people, and, in the context of media provoked parental anxiety, they draw on empirical studies about the actual risks and benefits. They also discuss the particular issues for children and young people who are "looked after" by public authorities and the need to balance concerns for Internet safety with access, digital literacy, and empowerment.

In the final chapter, LaMendola discusses the human encounter that constitutes the focus of human services by considering the concept of social presence in a networked society. Social presence is an aspect of human service which is taken for granted. The encounter between client and worker is at its heart. It is partly because of the perceived primacy of the interpersonal relationship for social work that theorists have sometimes been concerned about technologies displacing the human encounter. Many human service practitioners are also worried about the role of information systems, systems that may distort genuine human dialogue with a communication style driven by the need to feed the fields in a database. LaMendola addresses these concerns by deconstructing what is meant by the term social presence, whether face-to-face or mediated by technology, and articulating the key elements of "being present" to another. One consequence of his approach is to make problematic the quality of all kinds of social presence. While recognizing the inherent advantages of physical presence, he calls into question the assumption that physical presence is either necessary or sufficient for "social presence" to be felt, for a genuinely mutual human encounter to occur, or for a sense of community to be developed.

CONCLUSION

The chapters in this volume draw our attention, each in their own way, to connections of interest to the human services. Cinching a string around them is not our intention. In fact, they represent only a very small sample of the research emerging on human services in the context of the network society. Our hope is that in bringing together a collection of work from different human services domains – criminal justice, community care, and child welfare – we can draw attention to some common issues associated with the ways in which networked technologies are being harnessed for social purposes.

In a report surveying expert opinion on the influence of the Internet on the future of social relations, 85% agreed that the social benefits would far outweigh the negatives over the next decade (Anderson & Rainie, 2010). However, as Fischers' (1992) work suggests, the benefits of technology don't arise automatically, but are shaped by the influence of social actors. There is an opportunity for human service professionals to recognise their role in the social shaping of technology and to use their voice to promote social practices with technology that empowers people, sustains family life, and builds social capital. At the end of the day, promoting social welfare in the network society will not be a technological matter, it will be – as it always was – a moral and ethical one.

REFERENCES

Anderson, J.Q. & Rainie, L. (2010). *The Future of Social Relations*. Washington: Pew Internet & American Life Project. Retrieved from: http://pewinternet.org/Reports/2010/The-future-of-social-relations.aspx

Barbosa, L. (2009). *Uncovering the Hidden Web*. (Unpublished doctoral dissertation). The University of Utah, Salt Lake City, Utah.

Castells, M. (2000a). The Rise of the Network Society, the Information Age: Economy, Society and Culture Vol. I. (2nd ed). Cambridge, MA: Oxford, UK: Blackwell.

Cary, M. (2011). *Homeless turn to Twitter for food, shelter*. Retrieved from: http://www.cnn.com/2011/TECH/social.media/06/28/homeless.twitter.help/

Castells, M. (2004). The Power of Identity, the Information Age: Economy, Society and Culture Vol. II. (2nd ed). Cambridge, MA: Oxford, UK: Blackwell.

Castells, M. (2000b). End of Millennium, the Information Age: Economy, Society and Culture Vol. III. (2nd ed). Cambridge, MA: Oxford, UK: Blackwell.

charity: water (2011). Retrieved from: http://www.charitywater.org/http://www.charitywater.org/

Chou, S. W., Hunt, M. Y., Beckjord, B. E., Moser, P. R., & Hesse, W. B. (2009). Social Media Use in the United States: Implications for Health Communication. *Journal of Medical Internet Research, 11,* e48.

Cucciare, M. A., Weingardt, K. R., & Humphreys, K. (2009). How Internet technology can improve the quality of care for substance use disorders. *Current Drug Abuse Reviews, 2,* 256-262.

Cuijpers, P., Donker, T., van, S. A., Li, J., & Andersson, G. (2010). Is guided self-help as effective as face-to-face psychotherapy for depression and anxiety disorders? A systematic review and meta-analysis of comparative outcome studies. *Psychological Medicine,* 1-15.

Enos, G. (2008). Technology [online virtual platforms such as Second Life could help clients model recovery-affirming behaviors]. *Addict.Prof., 6,* 53-54.

Fischer, C.S. (1992). *America Calling: a social history of the telephone to 1940.* Berkeley: the University of California Press.

LaMendola, W. (1988). Networks and electronic communication. In B. Glastonbury, W. LaMendola, & S. Toole (Eds.), *Information Technology and the Human Services.* London: John Wiley & Sons.

LaMendola, W., Ballantyne, N., & Daly, E. (2009). Practitioner Networks: Professional Learning in the Twenty-First Century. *The British Journal of Social Work, 39*(4), 710-724.

LaMendola, W. (2011) Child Welfare & Technology. *CW360.* University of Minnesota: Center for Advanced Studies in Child Welfare. Spring, 2011.

McCluskey, U. (2005). To Be Met as a Person: the dynamics of attachment in professional encounters. London: Karnac Books.

Newman, M. G., Koif, D. F., Przeworski, A., & Llera, S. J. (2010). Anxiety disorders. In M.A.Cucciare & K. R. Weingardt (Eds.), *Using technology to support evidence-based behavioral health practices: A clinician's guide* (pp. 27-44). New York, NY, US: Routledge/Taylor & Francis Group.

Newman, M. G., Szkodny, L. E., Llera, S. J., & Przeworski, A. (2011). A review of technology-assisted self-help and minimal contact therapies for anxiety and depression: is human contact necessary for therapeutic efficacy? *Clinical Psychology Review, 31,* 89-103.

Putnam, R. D. (2000). Bowling Alone: the collapse and revival of American community. New York: Simon & Schuster.

United Nations (2011). *Report of the Special Rapporteur on the promotion and protection of the right to freedom of opinion and expression.* United Nations, General Assembly, Human Rights Council. Retrieved from: http://www2.ohchr.org/english/bodies/hrcouncil/docs/17session/A.HRC.17.27_en.pdf

VanDeMark, N.R., Burrell, N.R., LaMendola, W.F., Hoich, C.A., Berg, N.P., Medina, E. (2010). An exploratory study of engagement in a technology-supported substance abuse intervention. *Substance Abuse Treatment, Prevention, and Policy. Jun* 8;5:10.

Van Dijk, J. A. G. M. (1991). The Network Society: social aspects of new media. London: Sage.

Webb, L. T., Joseph, J., Yardley, L., & Michie, S. (2010). Using the Internet to Promote Health Behavior Change: A Systematic Review and Meta-analysis of the Impact of Theoretical Basis, Use of Behavior Change Techniques, and Mode of Delivery on Efficacy. *Journal of Medical Internet Research, 12,* e4.

Wellman, B. (2001). Physical place and cyber-place: The rise of networked individualism. *International Journal for Urban and Regional Research, 25,* 227–252.

Wilkinson, N., Ang, R. P., & Goh, D. H. (2008). Online video game therapy for mental health concerns: A review. *International Journal of Social Psychiatry, 54,* 370-382.

Yates, D. & Paquette, S. (2011). Emergency Knowledge Management and Social Media Technologies: A Case Study of the 2010 Haitian Earthquake. *International Journal of Information Management,* forthcoming.

Interoperability and the Future of Human Services

DICK SCHOECH

Arlington School of Social Work, Arlington, Texas

We are entering a period of interoperability in the human services, or the automatic global linking of information across different services and organizations. The purpose of this article is to get human service professionals to think about research, policy, management, and practice in a future service delivery system where data, information, and knowledge can be electronically exchanged and used globally. If human service professionals are to be intelligent discussants at the table when our future digital human services delivery infrastructure is planned, clear thinking about the practices, impacts, and issues of linking agency data globally is critical. Since the focus in this paper is on the impact of global data interchange, the difficult technical issues surrounding user authentication, security, and privacy are not discussed in the depth they require.

Interoperability is a term that is not commonly understood by most human service professionals, although most understand the trends that are making interoperability inevitable. In its simplest form, interoperability is the ability of electronically linked agencies to work together, to interoperate ("Interoperability," 2010). It has a technical component—data linking—and a practice component—the use of linked data in decision making. Formally, interoperability is defined as "the ability of two or more systems or components to exchange information and to use the information that has been exchanged" (Institute of Electrical and Electronics Engineers, 2005).

Interoperability is one of the most critical concepts facing the adoption and implementation of enhanced electronic information technologies into the health and human services.

Interoperability in the human services implies and involves the following concepts:

- Information from multiple agencies linked electronically to create one system from the user's perspective
- Electronic data interchange (EDI) or the automatic, instantaneous, seamless, and secure exchange of information between separate organizations based on predetermined data definitions, standards, and protocols
- Global sharing of proprietary information with user authentication and identity management tools to ensure data security, client privacy, and confidentiality
- Ways to meaningfully interpret the information exchanged; for example, common taxonomies, custom dashboards, ways to slice and dice and drill down into data to answer "what if" type of questions, data visualization techniques such as Online Analytic Processing (OLAP), visual maps for problem structuring and collaboration, etc. (Schoech, Fluke, Basham, Baumann, & Cochran, 2004; Horn & Weber, 2007)
- Local customization of standard practice processes, such as risk and safety assessments
- The potential for automated actions to be associated with information and analysis; for example, via intelligent agents, Web robots or bots, triggers, and alerts
- The use of open rather than proprietary standards for the free sharing of agency-owned information given each agency's restrictions on sharing
- Sets of tools and rules for encoding and transmitting documents to be exchanged, such as extensible markup language (XML) (O'Looney, 2005)
- Compliance with the Health Insurance Portability and Accountability Act (HIPAA) and other laws governing the sharing of health information in the United States and in other countries
- Standards for exchanging data from the World Wide Web Consortium (W3C) and other international organizations
- Systems that accumulate intelligence with use; for example, those using data mining, decision modeling, organizational intelligence strategies, wiki knowledge repositories, etc.

Historically, the real power of technological innovations is due to linking, through railroads, highway, telephone, and electric grid. Over the past 20 years, the linking of organizational information has been occurring in many segments of society (e.g., e-government). Therefore, we can expect it to happen in the human services. There is some evidence that the human services are beginning to enter this information-linking phase. One example is the homeless management information system (HMIS). HMIS is the result of a directive of the U.S. Congress to the Department of Housing and Urban Development (HUD) to gather data on homelessness and related services. HUD does not recommend specific HMIS software but provided communities with strategies and guidelines for selecting and implementing an HMIS (Center for Social Policy, 2003). Another example is the Prevention Management Reporting and Training System of the Substance Abuse and Mental Health Services Administration (SAMHSA) that provides three separate but integrated information services: (a) prevention resources, (b) data submissions, and (c) reporting services (https://www.pmrts.samhsa.gov/pmrts/Default.aspx). A final example is the AIDS Regional Information and Evaluation System (ARIES), which is a multistate system that helps providers automate, plan, manage, and report on client data (http://www.cdph.ca.gov/PROGRAMS/AIDS/Pages/OAARIESHome.aspx).

Several factors are driving this emerging global trend toward interconnectivity in the human services. First is the desire for more efficient (less costly) service delivery due to the need for services continually outstripping the supply in modern societies. Second is the push for more effective services by policymakers and especially by consumers and advocacy groups. Third is profit and influence; for example, many organizations such as Microsoft, Google, General Electric, and the Robert Woods Johnson Foundation have major efforts for automating health records. Electronic health records will spur many human services other than health to become interconnected. A fourth driving force is globalization, where local services are viewed as part of an international system of services. A fifth and final driving force is that businesses and governments are developing the tools and techniques for electronic information interchange, and these are filtering into all human services—see for example, Stewards of Change (2010) and State of Connecticut (Gordon, 2009). The difficulties in achieving interoperability are not primarily technical but concern the organizational and political changes that are required or that result from interoperability.

HUMAN SERVICE DELIVERY SYSTEM INFRASTRUCTURE AND INTEROPERABILITY

This article focuses on the development, use, and impact of an interoperable, global, human service delivery infrastructure (IGHI). A human service infrastructure can be defined as the arrangement and linkage of agencies, funding, technology, procedures, and people that support service delivery. One can take several different views of this infrastructure: a geographic location view, a financial view, an expertise view, or an information flow and use view. For this discussion, the information flow and use view will be defined as the interoperability model of the IGHI.

Ideally, the natural flow and use of agency information should not be modified by the use of technology. Rather, technology should be designed to reflect and support the natural information flows that agencies use to serve clients. While information flow and use should not be altered by technology, technology often offers agencies the opportunity to modify existing patterns of information flow and use in order to operate more efficiently.

Previous discussions of interoperability in the human services present a top-down model of information flow and use (O'Looney, 2005; Schoech, Fitch, MacFadden, & Schkade, 2002). This is partly because large government social service agencies are currently envisioning and implementing interoperability, such as the HMIS and other systems mentioned earlier. However, as technology advances, more distributed models of interoperability may be possible and desirable in order to accommodate how small, independent social service agencies handle and use information.

This section will compare and contrast three interoperability models. The first is a loose network of independent agencies illustrated by the concepts of cloud computing and smartphone apps. The second is a more formal network of small, independent organizations illustrated by interoperability in the travel industry. The third is a large organizational model illustrated by interoperability in the banking system. To heighten contrasts between the models and enhance understanding, model descriptions may be more stereotypic in this discussion than they are in reality. In addition, while pure models are presented, often a mix of models exists in various segments of societies.

Before discussing interoperability in human service agencies, it is useful to examine assumptions about the current human services delivery system in the United States and possibly in other developed countries. These are the following:

- Most agencies have personal computers, basic management oriented information systems, and Internet access for all staff. Agencies are struggling to keep the talent necessary to keep their systems up and running effectively, up to date with technology, and protected from threats posed by hackers, viruses, unauthorized access, and other security and privacy threats.
- In larger agencies, often data resides in antiquated legacy systems that serve their intended purpose but hinder interoperability because data are isolated in unlinked information silos.
- Most agency information systems are designed to serve the needs of managers rather than support frontline practitioners. Many critical decisions of frontline workers are based on information and knowledge that is not formally collected by most agencies.
- Practice knowledge is typically not automated but shared between professionals by face-to-face interactions or phone conversations with trusted colleagues. Experienced professionals have a large network of trusted colleagues whom they contact for help.

- Agencies often operate like small mom-and-pop organizations where quality control is based in people, not processes. We have all eaten at some mom-and-pop restaurants that were great, but we have also eaten at some that were bad. Sometimes even a great mom-and-pop restaurant can serve bad food, as when a novice cook substitutes for the chef who is out sick or off for the day.
- It is difficult to replicate a highly regarded mom-and-pop restaurant or human service because replication requires extracting expertise and processes from people and automating them.
- Clients often have very little knowledge of how services are delivered, and it is difficult for clients to find out this information.
- Convenience of services for clients is not a major concern when most agency services are designed. This is due to clients not having a choice. We know that if client choice exists, it drives service design. As with restaurants, people in most circumstances prefer convenience and known quality (e.g., fast food chains) to inconvenience and unknown quality (mom-and-pop restaurants).
- Few taxonomies exist for sharing information. For example, the meaning of the term client may vary by agency. Some agencies require a client to be one individual, while another may consider the family to be the client.
- Procedures for collecting, interpreting, and using data across agencies is rare, except at the top management and policy level of human service systems.

With these assumptions in mind, the next section presents three possible models for approaching interoperability in the human services.

Loosely Linked Network Model: Cloud Computing and Smart Phone Apps Example

DESCRIPTION OF THE MODEL

One model of agency information sharing that is beginning to emerge can be illustrated by software as a service (SaaS) and smart phone "apps" or applications. In this model, software is a service more than a product; that is, functionalities such as networking, storage, etc., are provided as needed using Web resources. Agencies acquire apps and tools that (a) reside and run locally on their agency system, (b) reside and run only on the Internet, or (c) reside locally and exchange information with multiple applications running on the Internet. These applications may be developed using tools like Webkit combined with HTML5 (Perlow, 2009).

In this model, each agency uses only the applications and tools needed to achieve their goals. Thus, the IGHI is an unstructured accumulation of tools, applications, standards, and taxonomies. The infrastructure may be similar to a social network such as Facebook, where multiple types and layers of connectivity exist between users. This model has the following characteristics:

- Provides information for services that is delivered on demand, just in time, and with user customization
- Lower overall infrastructure costs to agencies because only the applications and tools needed are used and systemwide activities are minimized
- Highly scalable and modular with connectivity and growth as needed
- Allows maximum agility and flexibility on the part of agencies

IMPACT ON PRACTICE

The impact on practice would be small and anticipated because agencies would buy into the larger infrastructure when needed and when they were ready. This model would give agencies and practitioners more control over the connectivity they desire and can afford. Internet based apps and tools would allow them to not only "Web enable" their systems but use the power offered by Web connectivity to the IGHI. An example of this model is the current automated health record where many corporate, private foundation, and government approaches exist ("NHS Connecting for Health," 2010).

ISSUES

Since this model contains no central infrastructure entities, the IGHI will have difficulty functioning because it lacks components such as quality control mechanisms. Apps that connect or coordinate with other apps might be needed, but these may be difficult to find due to the potential lack of agreed-on taxonomies, standardization, funding, and coordination. While this model may be the easiest to implement since less profound organizational changes are needed, the lack of a coordinating entity severely limits the benefits this model can provide in the long run.

Another issue relates to high overhead costs, due to inefficiencies, duplication, monopolies, etc. This is currently a problem with the U.S. health care system (or nonsystem as some point out) where administrative costs are higher and outcomes lower than more centralized systems providing the same services (Medicare and veterans health care).

This model suffers from the concept that a chain is only as strong as the weakest link. In this model, no entity has control over the quality of apps agencies use. This lack of control is especially problematic when trying to harden the IGHI against viruses, phishing attacks, and threats to data security, privacy, and confidentiality. Handling these threats is especially important since cloud computing puts the security of an agency's information in the hands of others beyond the agency's control and exposes it to global risk.

The recent coordinated attacks on the Google Gmail accounts of human rights activists illustrate the risks that exist when client records reside on or are linked to the Internet.

Network Model: Travel Industry Example

DESCRIPTION OF THE MODEL

The second interoperability model discussed is more formal in that central guidelines and standards have been established f0or entities to become part of the global infrastructure. An example can be seen by examining how interoperability has transformed the travel industry over the past 20 years. Some of the basic tasks of a travel agent are very similar to that of a social worker. One major set of tasks of a travel agency is to develop travel plans based on a traveler's needs and wants. A similar set of social work tasks is to develop an intervention plan based on a client's needs and wants. Contrasting how these tasks are handled illustrates the features of the network model of interoperability.

Twenty years ago, small independent mom-and-pop operations dominated the travel industry. When working with customers to develop their travel plans, travel agents used the telephone to find airline schedules, hotel availability, etc. Today, the interconnected information available to a travel agent has caused major changes in how travelers find vacations that meets their needs. Possible destinations, time restrictions, preferences, costs, etc., are entered into a Web application and the user is quickly presented with choices of destination, times, costs, accommodations, and other options. Many organizations worldwide, such as airlines, hotel chains, and rental car dealers, are linked via the Web during the planning process,. Some of these organizations use the information provided by the traveler to further their own goals. For example, immediately after the traveler makes an airline reservation on a travel site, the information can be used by an airline application that optimizes airline profits by ensuring that each plane is full with the highest paying passengers. Based on a number of optimization criteria, subsequent travelers booking the same flight may pay more for a similar ticket to the same destination.

Now consider the technology typically used when clients want to find a counseling service that meets their needs. Clients can call 211, if implemented in their area, to obtain a list of possible agencies to contact. 211 callers may be transferred to an agency or be required to call each agency separately. A receptionist, with little or no computer support, usually handles these calls. Each agency screens clients in or out of its particular services rather than into a service delivery system that is integrated to meet client needs. No human service IT (information technology) applications analyze the client's problem and preferences and use the results to find several good service options. No applications exist to optimize an agency's goals by screening clients in or out based on the matching of client needs and worker expertise, the number of services the agency has available, or client outcome expectations.

This comparison, which is illustrated in Table 1, shows that human services agencies, which often make life-changing or even life and death decisions for people in need, lag behind business use of IT, even businesses providing routine recreational services. Table 1 also shows the potential

TABLE 1 Interoperability Characteristics Relevant for a Travel Agent and a Social Worker

Travel agent task of assessment and trip planning	Social worker task of assessment and service planning
Concerns inconsequential tasks in terms of a person's life.	Concerns tasks varying from inconsequential to those critical to survival in society, assessment of risk due to child abuse.
Involves an infrastructure with high levels of information flows and use between system components.	Involves many separate agencies with little data exchanged.
Web application works a traveler through the screening process.	Some Web IT screening applications may exist, but most information collected from client is used by managers, not workers.
Work processes are driven by quick access to data in multiple databases of many organizations, such as airlines, hotels, rentals, and tours.	Work processes are people based; that is, most information is obtained from a worker's informal network of colleagues.
Consistent, automatic, systemwide updating and forecasting (e.g., airplane passenger load optimization).	Sharing of information and expertise results in uneven quality (e.g., high quality such as when a practitioner makes a personal referral to a colleague or poor quality where the client is given a list of agencies to contact for services).
Most knowledge resides in the system.	Most knowledge resides in people.
It is easy to start up a new service and become part of the system.	It is easy to start up a new agency but no "system" to link into.
System allows travelers to set up e-mail alerts that are triggered by data (e.g., price changes).	Clients rarely can set triggers that alert them with important information.
Service excellence and convenience are key issues with substantial data collected from travelers to optimize quality.	Agency convenience often dominates service decisions with little client follow up data available for optimizing service quality.
Services supplemented by confirming e-mails and self-help Web sites; for example, educational Web sites, blogs, ratings by previous travelers, RSS (Really Simple Syndication) feeds, etc.	Infrequent use of confirming e-mails, educational and self-help Web sites, and quality ratings from previous clients.
Travelers' data is retained on an as-needed basis with few regulations covering data retention and interchange.	Data is often retained for long periods of time and subject to many laws and regulations (e.g., HIPAA).

for using current interoperability technology to improve the IGHI and, consequently, the services delivered to agencies connected to this infrastructure.

IMPACT ON PRACTICE

Connecting travel agents to a global interoperable infrastructure has dramatic impacts; for example, most travel agents have lost their jobs in the past 20 years. People wanting to travel use Web sites operated by large corporations (Travelocity, Expedia) that have the resources to develop a robust travel site capable of performing all of the tasks of a travel agent in a small mom-and-pop organization along with many new tasks travelers appreciate. Most travel sites educate the traveler about potential destinations, provide reviews and comments by previous customers, and offer special pricing on hotels and rental cars. Another impact is that the traveler has much more control of quality and service due to competition. Travel Web sites compete on ease of use, convenience, service quality, customer education, and flexibility during the interaction. Components of the travel industry are linked depending on the needs of the system to provide quality services. Some links may be very loose, such as links to information about national parks. Some links may be tightly integrated, such as when a traveler books a flight and the airline uses that booking to adjust the prices for the next customer based on an automatic computer model that optimizes loads and profits. Some travel sites can send out alerts based on triggers; for example, you might set a trigger to send you an e-mail alert if the price of a vacation package decreases to fit your budget. Travelers see the many interconnected travel services as one system and are unaware of the complex connectivity that occurs as they interact with the site.

ISSUES

The loosely coupled network model illustrates many issues that human service agencies must address as they struggle with interoperability. The major issue is how to make a globally connected system out of many independent local agencies. Our current system reflects the independence of funding sources, professionals, and system managers who have little incentive to develop an IGHI. However, some major governmental funding sources are beginning to see that categorical funding of services has produced a system in which client choice and service quality are not key factors in service delivery design. Recent initiatives mentioned previously may break this strangle hold that financing has on system design, thus allowing more integrated, coordinated, and client centered service delivery.

Another major issue eluded to in the previous discussion concerns the automation of routine, repetitive tasks. Travel companies found it cost-beneficial to capture and automate the knowledge possessed by travel agents. Some of knowledge social workers possess to perform routine job tasks can be automated, leaving workers to perform more complex, integrative tasks such as assessment and intervention design. Thus, worker education and training might need to focus on the complex integrative tasks that defy automation. Automation makes our lack of understanding of the knowledge base of social work a major issue.

A final issue concerns protecting privacy and confidentiality. One big difference presented in Table 1 is that human service agencies must often hold sensitive data for long periods of time, and they need to meet the demands of growing statutory data protection legislation. Large networked systems will need to handle these data so that human service professionals will trust that client data are secure and privacy and confidentiality are protected as services are interconnected and data shared. Clients are often so eager to get services that they minimize the necessity of privacy and security protection. Clients often only show concern once their privacy or confidentiality has been violated. Client advocacy groups, however, are often in a position to understand the issues of security and privacy and can help balance them with access, legal, and service quality issues.

Top-Down Model: Banking Industry Example

Description of the Model

Changes in banking over the past 20 years illustrate a third model of interoperability that is common in the corporate sectors of society. Twenty years ago, local banks manually mailed checks and currencies around the world. Today, a global banking infrastructure exists with EDI protected by numerous authentication, privacy, and confidentiality safeguards. People can pay bills using the Internet or obtain local currency using an ATM (automated teller machine) almost anywhere in the world. Sophisticated computer programs, called agents or bots, analyze financial information for "unusual activity" and trigger the sending of alerts. For example, some banks alert customers of large credit card purchases originating far from their home.

Although it is a simplification, we can point to three major components of the global banking infrastructure: (a) local bank branch offices (e.g., your local Bank of Scotland), (b) networks of banks (e.g., Lloyds Banking Group of which the Bank of Scotland is a part), and (c) a global consortium for coordinating and monitoring international banking (e.g., International Monitory Fund). Local banks that chose not to connect to this global infrastructure have gone out of business. This quiet banking revolution was driven by customers who gravitated to banks that offered a variety of convenient, reliable, and quick services.

When viewed from the perspective of the top-down model, the three components of the IGHI will be: (a) local agencies (e.g., a local Red Cross agency), (b) affiliations of local agencies (such as a group of community agencies providing Red Cross type services that are interested in sharing information), and (c) a global consortium for accumulating knowledge and developing protocols (e.g., the International Federation of Red Cross and Red Crescent Societies and its designated U.S. affiliate the American Red Cross). These three components constitute an information-sharing infrastructure, not an organizational or service structure. The extent of information sharing, the extent of adherence to protocols, and the latitude of agencies to "do their own thing" within the infrastructure will be continually negotiated between agency administrators, professional associations, funding sources, and community stakeholders, including client advocates.

IMPACT ON PRACTICE

While local agencies connected to the IGHI will seem the same to clients, their operations that support management and workers will be quite different. The affiliate of local agencies can perform many routine tasks such as scheduling intra-agency meetings, sifting through volumes of information from multiple agencies to construct client service histories, collecting evidence on client progress, and keeping everyone informed on data security, privacy, and confidentiality threats. With many routine tasks automated, social workers can concentrate on high-level tasks such as assessment, which includes observation, sensing, forming relationships, displaying empathy, working through "what if" scenarios, and making complex judgments and cognitive leaps. Local social workers can also contribute to the global knowledge base by online involvement with global expert teams to research complex problem. While movement toward the top-down model of interoperability might be slow due to the required changes in services and agencies, over the next 20 years this model of interoperability will have a profound influence on social work practice.

ISSUES

The recent collapse of the global banking system illustrates that newly designed infrastructures can have unforeseen problems. The failure to modernize and enforce regulations allowed many banks to take excessive risks that sacrificed long-term goals for short-term gain. What made good short-term sense for certain components of the banking system was not good for the total banking system. Agencies must work together to achieve *concerted suboptimization* in which each entity of a system must often sacrifice and function suboptimally to achieve systemwide goals. Without systemwide monitoring and control, organizations that ignore guidelines or exploit loopholes for their own benefit can threaten the survival of the total system. Lack of agencies working as a team to support systemwide goals can be a major issue. Without self-correcting mechanisms in place, new and redesigned systems are vulnerable to manipulations by subsystems to maximize their benefits and power at the expense of the larger system. The IGHI will swing back and forth between too much control and too much freedom by member agencies. As the infrastructure matures, these swings should be less dramatic and failures less visible and damaging.

Another issue mentioned previously concerns information security and privacy protection. Since the top-down infrastructure has more controls and continuous quality improvement (CQI) activities, this model will be more attractive to governmental and large social service delivery system that value accountability over flexibility, efficiency, and effectiveness.

DISCUSSION

Connectivity technology is progressing rapidly, so models other than the three discussed in this article may emerge. In addition, different communities and different human service areas will have different approaches to interoperability, so some communities may have a mixture of all three models. The loosely linked network may be a beginning model because it requires the least conceptual and organizational change and allows agencies to move gradually from being completely independent to linked entities. Linking stages may emerge; for example, nonthreatening apps like shared calendars and information and referral systems tasks may be linked first. These first linked tasks may be those that are high volume, routine, repetitive, and require extensive paperwork. These are exactly the low-level task that human service professionals loathe. The network model may be an intermediate model and more common in service areas that are more decentralized in funding and services, such as aging and addictions. Eventually, interoperability might favor the top-down model, especially in large systems such as child welfare and health. However, it may take a while for agencies to see themselves as needing to be an integral part of an IGHI.

Whatever model or mix of models exists, the need exists for three sets of "players." These three are local agencies linked to the infrastructure, local networks of agencies, and globally networked think tanks. Each of these will be discussed, along with the required attitude and organizational changes required.

Local Agencies

At the local agency level, the attitude and systematic changes necessary for interoperability to occur are as follows:

- Processed information is seen as a key resource for staff at all levels of an agency.

- Staff are receptive to technology guided practice and should be encouraged to use facts rather than attitudes to skeptically challenge IT guidance.
- The agency is viewed as an integral part of a national or global infrastructure.
- Change in work patterns should be accepted so that technology that is developed nationally and globally can be customized to support local routine tasks such as scheduling meetings and constructing client records by linking to the databases of multiple agencies.
- Services are not viewed as unique but as sharing many processes capable of being supported by customizing global information and knowledge.
- Staff value adding local expertise to the knowledge base of the larger system, such as having highly skilled local workers join national and international teams researching how best to work difficult cases.

Most local agencies desire access to client information that other agencies possess. They usually have less desire to share their client information with other agencies. Currently, the benefits of not sharing are often greater than the benefits of sharing client information. Costs to share information are relatively easy to calculate, while the impact of shared information on the quality of services is difficult to calculate. In addition, most agency information systems support managers, not frontline workers who most need multiagency information. Finally, the overhead costs associated with connectivity and being part of a larger system is a disincentive. As indicated earlier, agencies might be receptive to linking to other agencies if they see their chances of continued funding increase. Since financial incentives have been important in encouraging interoperability in other segments of society, the categorical nature of human services funding and the lack of client choice may result in the human services interoperability taking longer than in other sectors.

Affiliations of Local Agencies

The local network of agencies provides some or all of the following functions:

- Support IT operations and information system development
- Negotiate/maintain agreements on data sharing between agencies
- Develop multiagency ways to measure and monitor client process and outcomes
- Interpret and customize global knowledge to local situations
- Customize "alerts" and "triggers" for local practices and politics using multiagency data
- Maintain quality control systems and mechanisms (e.g., mechanisms for exception monitoring)

- Help agencies develop and apply tools and techniques to ensure information security and privacy compliance (e.g., conform to HIPAA requirements)

Communities often have a group of technology savvy agency professionals who meet periodically to discuss how to use technology to better coordinate and improve service delivery. Some members of this group may be connected to federal or state information sharing networks, such as the homeless information system mentioned previously. This local group often struggles as it has little or no formal authority and responsibility due to local agencies seeking to remain independent and not seeing the need for empowering a local infrastructure. However, some multiagency human services may encourage and sponsor this group (e.g., the United Way) as its role becomes more important in managing interoperability at the local level.

Globally Networked Think Tanks

The national/global think tank or institute component of the IGHI provides some or all of the following functions:

- Develops taxonomies for sharing data that conform to WC3 and XML standards and guidelines
- Develops measures, standards, and data sets for determining service quality and acknowledging the cultural context of practice in various locales
- Accumulates repositories of research, best practices, stories/practice wisdom, etc., for system learning, especially as the current group of baby boomer practitioners retire and leave an expertise gap in some agencies
- Conducts decision modeling, forecasting, data mining of large datasets, meta-analyses, pattern recognition, prediction, etc., for critical problems facing groups of similar agencies
- "Pushes out" diagnosis, prognosis, predictions, proven interventions, best practices, etc., to agencies when they need them and in the format they need them (e.g., in Web based structured processes that novices can follow)
- Maintains open standards and open source alternative tools so that agencies are not locked into proprietary systems
- Convenes pools of experts to guide and vet research, practice techniques, lessons learned, changing work patterns, etc., on various topics so that agencies and their stakeholders understand that the move toward interconnectivity is a move toward service quality
- Provides technical support with knowledge sharing tools like wikis, content management systems such as Drupals, and collaborative tools such as Basecamp

- Provide guidance on win-win brokering of information, since information is power and it is easy to get caught in win-lose connectivity scenarios that alienate those left out of the move toward an IGHI
- Develops informational Web sites and self-help interventions for common, structured problems, such as information and referral and the treatment of mild cases of phobias, addictions, anxiety, etc.

No matter which interoperability model dominates the future IGHI, a national and global research think tank function is needed. This is because many issues are beyond the capacity of local agencies to solve and because agencies can learn and adapt what others have found to be successful. The function is not to "manage" but to support, link, provide expertise, and research applications that involve risks that agencies cannot take on their own. Accumulating knowledge repositories to support practice is especially important as social workers are increasingly hired on a contract basis to perform diverse tasks with very little training and technical support (e.g., homebound case management). These repositories are also important for Internet savvy clients who have the capacity to search out information on their problem and its solution (e.g., WebMD). A related task concerns information literacy and helping practitioners and clients assess the accuracy of information found on the Web.

In order for the social work profession to be a key player in developing the IGHI, much research needs to be conducted on a global basis. For example, XML taxonomies are needed to allow for automated data interchange. Standards and techniques are needed for client authentication, privacy, and confidentiality. Work is beginning in these areas, such as by the child welfare XML Work Group and by United Way of America. However, this work is underresourced and not global in nature. Global human services organizations capable of carrying out the think tank function do not exist. In addition, most funding sources for human services IT are local rather than global. In the business sector, cost savings due to increased efficiency and productivity fund IT infrastructure research and development. However, the current financing of human services does not encourage IGHI funding.

CONCLUSIONS

Throughout history, technologies that provide linking and connectivity have had a substantial impact on most segments of society. The human services, which are dominated by many unconnected agencies and services, will follow other segments of society in linking organizational information and using linked information to support practice. This linking will develop slowly due to categorical funding for many services and due to the organizational and work pattern changes that are required. While the overall vision of interoperability is relatively easy to identify, the path for our unconnected human services to move toward an IGHI remains unclear. This article presented and discussed three possible models of interoperability that can be seen as three stages of interoperability progression. Additional research and thinking needs to examine service areas and communities where interoperability has begun so we can learn from our mistakes. In the end, the IGHI will have a profound impact on human service delivery. Human service professionals need to understand interoperability processes and tools so that they can be involved in their development. Interoperability is too important to be developed by business managers, IT technicians, or politicians without the expertise that human service professionals have to offer.

REFERENCES

Center for Social Policy. (2003). Homeless management information system (HMIS) consumer guide: A review of available HMIS solutions. Retrieved from http://www.disasterhousing.gov/offices/cpd/homeless/hmis/assistance/consumerguide/toc.pdf

Gordon, E. (2009). Lessons from across the country. Retrieved from http://www.ct.gov/oca/lib/oca/human_services_presentation_5–27–09_final.ppt

Horn, E. R., & Weber, R. P. (2007). New tools for resolving wicked problems: Mess mapping and resolution mapping processes. Retrieved from http://www.strategykinetics.com/files/New_Tools_For_Resolving_Wicked_Problems.pdf

Institute of Electrical and Electronics Engineers. (2005). Standards dictionary: Glossary of terms & definitions. Retrieved from http://www.ieeeusa.org/policy/POSITIONS/NHINinteroperability.html#_ftn1

Interoperability. (2010). Wikipedia. Retrieved from http://en.wikipedia.org/wiki/Interoperability

NHS connecting for health. (2010). Retrieved from http://www.connectingforhealth.nhs.uk/

O'Looney, J. (2005). Social work and the new semantic information revolution. *Administration in Social Work, 29*(4), 5–34.

Perlow, J. (2009). For vertical market smartphone apps, is Webkit the "true" dev target? Retrieved from http://blogs.zdnet.com/perlow/?p=11744&tag=nl.e539

Schoech, D., Fitch, D., MacFadden, R., & Schkade, L. L. (2002). From data to intelligence: Introducing the intelligent organization, *Administration in Social Work, 26*(1), 1–21.

Schoech, D., Fluke, J., Basham, R., Baumann, D., & Cochran, G. (2004). Visualizing multilevel agency data using OLAP technology: An illustration & lessons learned. *Journal of Technology in Human Services, 22*(4), 93–111.

Stewards of Change. (2010). InterOptimability: Connecting systems by optimizing outcomes. Retrieved from http://www.stewardsofchange.com/Consulting/Pages/InterOptimability.aspx

Eternal Vigilance Inc.: The Satellite Tracking of Offenders in "Real Time"

MIKE NELLIS

Glasgow School of Social Work, Glasgow, Scotland

The satellite tracking of offenders, particularly sex offenders, has grown in significance in the United States since the late 1990s. Some evaluations have been undertaken, but few of the larger theoretical questions it raises, as an aspect of surveillance and remote location monitoring, have been explored. Drawing in part on the work of Manuel Castells and Paul Virilio and on the concept of "time–space compression," this paper appraises the significance of satellite tracking in the context of "the network society" and assesses its implications for supervising offenders in so-called "real time." It speculates on the different temporal experiences of monitors and the monitored and explores a dubious but possible future development in tracking technology: the power to inflict pain at a distance, forms of which were in fact considered by the those who first imagined offender tracking in the 1970s. For some offenders, potentially subject to lifelong satellite tracking, the specter of "eternal vigilance" is raised, and the paper concludes with ethical questions this practice provokes.

INTRODUCTION

In the software universe of light-speed travel, space may be traversed literally in "no-time"; the difference between far away and down here is cancelled. Space no more sets limits to action and its effects, and counts for little, or does not count at all.

—Bauman (2000, p. 17)

Mobile communication and locatability technologies—some audio, some visual, some simulated, or permutations of all three—are now commonly being used to provide immediate and constant information to a range of law enforcement and correctional agencies. These enable "real time" data sharing between street-level operatives and control centers or "back offices," accelerating and affecting decisions in both places. Even as shrewd a judge of evolving control technologies as William Burroughs did not quite see "real time" mobile communication coming, nor did he appraise its implications for crime control: "control," he wrote matter-of-factly in the 1960s, "needs time in which to exercise control" (Burroughs, 1986, p. 117). True enough, even now, but the time span is lessening. The satellite tracking of offenders, on which this paper will focus, involves micromanaging the specific locations and schedules of offenders over short or sustained periods of time, sometimes (but not always) in "real time." Potentially, this adds an unprecedented element of reach and immediacy to the supervision of offenders in the community, pinpointing a mobile offender's whereabouts, enabling remote communication (by phone or text) with him or her, and making schedule violations more certain of rapid detection than ever before. While there remains, for now, a crucial difference between remotely *knowing* in "real time" and being able (as a crime controller) to remotely *act* in "real time," it is indisputable that late modern, especially 21st century, communication and locatability technologies have already refined and modulated the temporality of crime control in significant—and probably unfinished—ways (Lyon, 2006; Genosko & Thompson, 2006).

Satellite tracking, using the Global Positioning System (GPS), extends the earlier and still dominant form of remote radio frequency (RF) electronic monitoring used with offenders, that of house arrest, which became widespread in the United States in the 1980s and Europe in the 1990s (Lilly, 1992; Monmonier, 2004). The tracking of offender movements had in fact been imagined before the monitoring of single offender locations came into being, in the 1960s, albeit not using satellites, but in practice it emerged partly as a response to the perceived limitations of "mere" house arrest. Advances in GPS technology enabled penal applications of it in the late 1990s, and on any given day in the United States in 2009 some 44,000 offenders were subject to it, mostly sex offenders released from prison (Button, DeMichelle, & Payne 2009). It was piloted in England and Wales in 2004–2006 but not deemed cost-effective (Shute, 2007). It is used on a small scale—less than 100 people combined—in France and the Netherlands (Elzinga & Nijboer, 2006), while in South Korea (by mid-2009) more than

500 sex offenders have been subject to it. While still small scale, it may yet become more prevalent in the United States and internationally (Doffing, 2010), and this paper will tentatively explore its implications as a form of "real time" crime control.

TIME–SPACE COMPRESSION AND THE NETWORK SOCIETY

Satellite tracking is a vivid example of "time–space compression" in penal practice. Globe-spanning computerized information and communication technologies have wrought something akin to "the death of distance" in the late modern world, making it possible to synchronize certain types of action in places that are far apart from one another. The availability of instant/immediate knowledge about remote events then alters our perception of what "now" means, disembedding its traditional association with "here," enabling us to share a "real time" experience of "now" with someone who may be geographically distant, possibly with a correspondingly reduced awareness of one's own immediate social and physical surroundings. The existential sense of rootedness, of boundedness within a particular time and place, can be displaced partially, if not completely by a sense of simultaneous connection to "elsewhere." A remotely monitored offender who knows that his present location can be pinpointed and that his past locations can be traced may sense behavioral constraints on him that his unmonitored predecessors would not have experienced.

The sociotechnical process of "time–space compression" is not new. As Barbara Adam (2004) writes, "Much of the history of technology can be read as advances in speed" (p. 129), of transport, production, and communication, all largely in pursuit of productivity and profit. Management strategies throughout the 20th century sought ever more efficient uses of time and the reduction of unnecessary delay. Taylorism aimed to shrink production processes to the minimum of time, energy, and motion required. Post-Fordism valorized "just-in-time" production, tied to ever more precise anticipation/stimulation of the time and place of demand. Urban theorist Paul Virilio (1997, 2006) subsequently added important political dimensions to established economic explanations of speed, arguing that "speed machines" and "vision machines" and most recently "optoelectronics" have always been integral to the achievement and maintenance of governmental domination in any given territory, whether by the movement of armies, the velocity of weapons, or, nowadays, the range and intensity of electronic surveillance. I will draw on Virilio's work later in this paper.

Manuel Castells's (1996; Castells, Fernandez-Ardevol, Qiu, & Aey, 2006) work has arguably been the most influential in this field. Close interconnections between politics, commerce, and culture inform his conceptualization of "the network society," a society to whose organization "micro-electronic based information and communication technologies" are structurally constitutive. His account is grounded firmly in the changes that took place in capitalism in the last quarter of the 20th century. First, global financial markets were transformed by deliberate policies of deregulation, new computerized information technologies, and new management techniques, and for the "first time in history" (in the 1990s) worked in real time, with "capital [being] shuttled back and forth between economies in a matter of hours, minutes and sometimes seconds" (Castells, 1996, p. 467). Second, newly emerged global multimedia networks made possible "instant information throughout the globe, mixed with live reporting from across the neighborhood, providing unprecedented temporal immediacy to social events and cultural expressions" (p. 491). The advent of the Internet, of cyberspace, and of mobile phone technology extended and individualized the possibility of "real time" communication to millions of people, whether in short bursts (texting) or more total immersion (online gaming, social networking sites, Second Life).

The cumulative cultural and psychological consequence of these recent sociotechnical developments has been the shortening of durational expectancies, an emergent sense that events and processes (economic, managerial, and political) should and could happen faster than hitherto. In the resultant sensibility, immediacy and instantaneity become mental ideals against which even mundane actions in the real world are subconsciously measured (Tomlinson, 2007). "Time is compressed, and ultimately denied in culture [itself], as a primitive replica of the fast turnover in production, consumption, ideology and politics on which our society is based" (Castells, 1996, p. 493). In extremis, the compression of time produces what William Bogard (1996) presciently called "the telematic imaginary"—a technophiliac dream that action at a distance (remote control) by state/corporate agencies will one day be a commonplace means of creating and sustaining social and political order. He subsequently acknowledged that while the dream itself does stimulate the development of technologies that aspire toward its realization, their actual impact in practice should not be exaggerated. What actually emerge are

> real and imperfect strategies of extending social control beyond systems of confinement, deterritorialising the space of enclosure, allowing enclosure to operate, as it were, "at a distance," or rather without regard to distance, the model of *telematic or virtual confinement*. The classic example is the monitoring bracelets worn by sex offenders to track their movements outside the prison, but it is easy to think of even more radical devices such as genetic mitigations and implants . . . what we are witnessing is a kind of dematerialisation of control. (Bogard, 2006, p. 71)

While "dematerialization" captures something of the "invisibility" of telematic controls, it is important not to lose sight of the very real material context—the infrastructures and hardware—in which these developments are grounded. Castells accurately describes the "new organizational forms" that create ineluctable pressures for instantaneity and immediacy. He has in mind commercial organizations, but they could just as easily be state bureaucracies and in particular crime control agencies such as the police or probation and parole services. They exhibit

> flexible forms of management, relentless utilisation of fixed capital, intensified performance of labor strategic alliances, interorganisational linkages, all come down to shortening time per operation and to speeding up turnover of resources. Indeed, the just-in-time inventory management procedures has been the symbol of lean production [although]...it belongs to a pre-electronic age of manufacturing technology. (Castells, 1996, p. 467)

Castells questions the aptness of the term "real time," preferring "network time" to denote an array of different points (nodes) in a digital network in simultaneous communication with one another, thereby creating a shared "now." He distinguishes "network time" from the sequential and rhythmic time that we experience "naturally," in particular social locations, when we are not connected electronically to anywhere else. "Network time" never fully displaces people's experience of time as sequence and rhythm, but to a greater or lesser degree it superimposes a new layer of temporal experience on their lives, whose meaning and significance to an individual's sense of identity varies according to age, occupation, and class. Many organizations require their employees to be extensively immersed in it, in constant communication with counterparts around the country or the globe, ensuring that it becomes part of their work identity.

GPS TECHNOLOGY, COMMERCE, AND PENAL INNOVATION

The Global Positioning System (GPS) is one of the communication technologies that underpin Castells's (1996, p. 3) conception of the "network society." It is a satellite-based navigation system created by the U.S. military in 1974 for their own use and extended to commercial, civilian (and other governmental), uses in the 1980s. It relies on 24 solar-powered satellites orbiting 12,000 miles above the earth, four of which are notionally "visible" at any one time from any terrestrial location. A portable GPS receiver can triangulate light speed signals from the satellites to determine latitude, longitude, and altitude, information that "can then be displayed graphically on a map" (Buck, 2009, p. 2), locating a person or object in "real time" to within a matter of meters. Tiny wavers in the satellites' orbits, the particular geometric alignment of the four "visible" ones, atmospheric conditions, and tall buildings can still affect the quality and accuracy of GPS pinpointing.

Even with four satellites, the relatively weak signal strength available to civilian users means that "GPS units often do not work indoors, underwater or underground" (Buck, 2009, p. 3). As general demand for "location-based services" has grown, various ways have been developed to address these limitations; both assisted GPS (A-GPS) and Advanced Forward Link Trilateration (AFLT) link to the cellular radio network to fill in the gaps when GPS is not available, on both of which U.S. criminal justice has capitalized (Buck, 2009b).

In general, "commercial applications of GPS far exceed those of the military...the private sector continues to use GPS in ways that the original developers could never have imagined" (Benshoof, 2007, p. 147). Customizing GPS technology as a penal measure is one such application, although in this context "military" and "penal" uses are not epistemologically or institutionally distinct: GPS tracking exemplifies what Haggerty and Erickson (2001) see as the increasing infusion of "military technoscience" into criminal justice. It emerged in the late 1990s as (in part) a solution to the high financial cost of imprisonment and as a means of making the supervision of offenders much tougher—more regulatory, more onerous—than anything probation officers could have managed (Moore & Thurston, 2009). Tracking built on the first forms of electronic monitoring (EM), which used remote location monitoring technology to enforce house arrest (curfews), pinpointing an offender's presence or absence from a single designated location for so many hours per day (often, but not always overnight), for so many weeks, months, or years (Stacey, 1995). The process by which a penal crisis—the effect of excessive imprisonment on many U.S. state budgets was proving catastrophic in respect of other public services—calls forth a new technological response, is beyond the scope of this paper, but there were entrepreneurs and "imagineers" in both government and the commercial world who sensed an opportunity (Nellis, 2006, 2009a, 2009b). Public safety concerns about released prisoners, especially those convicted of sexual violence to children, were simultaneously producing demands for more controlling measures than conventional parole, and GPS satellite tracking seemed to offer precisely this. By following movement on a 24/7/365 basis it could generate more data for supervisors. By enabling "exclusion zones" it could better protect former or prospective victims, and by creating "inclusion zones" (workplace, treatment center or one's own home) it could replicate EM house arrest. By constantly reminding offenders that their locations were known and/or traceable, that their pattern of movement could be "profiled" and nefarious intent inferred, and that their compliance with temporal schedules could always be checked, it seemed plausible that GPS tracking would enhance deterrence and reduce crime (International Association of Chiefs of Police, 2008).

While decisions to introduce satellite tracking schemes are political (and economic, spurred by the need to reduce burgeoning prison costs by facilitating structured early release programs), the role of commercial organizations in promoting electronic monitoring in general and satellite tracking in particular cannot be discounted. A global "commercial-corrections complex," rooted in but not exclusive to the United States, has emerged out of the old security industry to encompass the building and running of private prisons and, more recently, the telecommunication applications underpinning EM (Lilly & Deflem, 1996; Lilly & Knepper, 1993; Christie, 2000; Paterson, 2007a). Some of the organizations involved are indigenous U.S. companies, and others are global corporations. Some simply sell monitoring technologies to law enforcement and correctional agencies, while others sell more sophisticated computerized case management packages that include the technologies. All emphasize the cutting edge nature of their contributions to crime control, marketing their product as a modernizing technology, offering more total oversight of offenders to correctional agencies than has hitherto been possible. "Leap into the future," invites Shadowtrack, whose program "couples interactive voice response technology and voice biometrics authentication to keep track of offenders via the most modern and flexible telephone solutions available"

Surveys undertaken in the United States by the *Journal of Electronic Monitoring* in 2002–2003 and 2008–2009 indicate that the number of companies involved in GPS tracking has grown significantly. ProTech and iSECUREtrac were alone in the early period. By the later period they had been joined by some of the older EM companies (BI Incorporated, ElmoTech [an Israeli company with a global presence], G4S Justice Services, and Serco Geograpfix) and some new GPS companies (Satellite Tracking of People [STOP], Corrections Services, Digital Technologies 2000, ActSoft Inc., Guidance Monitoring Ltd, Alert System Corporation, and Omnilink Inc.) (*Journal of Offender Monitoring*, 2009). These companies (or at least their GPS arms) come into being because they sense a market emerging. They do not create the market as such but by their presence (and advertising) they shape it, highlighting the limitations of existing crime control systems by promoting something "better," stimulating professional (and managerial) imaginations, and expanding governmental horizons as to what is possible (Nellis, 2009b).

Perusal of the images and language in the various companies' advertisements is revealing. The notion of *incessance*, knowing where offenders are in real or near-real time over sustained periods (and being able to record and retrieve this data), is integral to them. It is the key selling point that makes GPS tracking superior to mere house arrest versions of EM. More especially it is what makes GPS tracking so much more protective of the public than mere probation or parole, whose one-to-one, face-to-face contact with offenders, however systematic and orderly, was at best intermittent and mostly undertaken during daytime hours. iSECUREtrac, for example, plays directly on the limitations of *mere* nighttime curfew tagging: after headlining with "Do you know your offenders are compliant when they're way from home? We check every 10 seconds!" they follow through with:

> iSECUREtrac GPS systems offer you the truth. You can hold your offenders accountable to the places they've been and the times they've been there, 24/7/365, anywhere in the world. Additionally GPS tracking systems can greatly increase your level of offender supervision without adding to officer workload. iSECUREtrac alone can provide you with location and compliance verification every 10 seconds, fastest violation reporting on the market, user-friendly, yet powerful, web-based software; proven GPS policies and best practice for agencies.

Syscon's case management system emphasizes automation over real-time monitoring but nonetheless lays great stress on the sense that everything pertinent to supervision is being taken care of (incessantly, by machines). Their advertisement, featuring a sleeping man with a contented look on his face, seeks to dispel anxieties about offenders' nighttime activities:

> This probation officer is using Syscon's automated systems to manage his low risk caseload with a range of kiosk, voice recognition and GPS technologies handling report-ins, the collection of fines, fees and restitution, and secure monitoring—all wrapped up in a fully integrated system. Only Syscon can offer you the full service package from end to end. It is no wonder he sleeps easy. (*Journal of Offender Monitoring*, 2009)

Despite the pitch of this particular advertisement, it is worth noting that automated data collection technologies generate an excess of information that requires *additional* labor time to process (International Association of Chiefs of Police, 2008).

THE PRACTICE OF SATELLITE TRACKING

In essence, the GPS tracking of offenders involves a group of staff in a monitoring center, who may be police or probation officers (or civilian staff in either agency) or employees of commercial organizations contracted to provide a service to probation, who sit at computer screens monitoring the movements of offenders, checking compliance with supervision requirements, periodically speaking by phone or text to the offenders, and processing and recording the data that emerges from this. The monitoring center may be hundreds of miles from where the offenders under surveillance live, and—if this is a commercial enterprise—far from where the probation or police officers work. Such monitoring center staff may have no direct knowledge of the neighborhoods in which the people they are tracking live; all they see are maps and data on a screen. Monitoring centers are usually staffed on a shift system, to ensure 24/7/365, "round the clock" cover. Their staff can contact law enforcement or correctional officials to inform them of what their offenders are doing, or, in respect of nighttime incidents, can leave them messages that they pick up the following morning.

While certain features and principles are common to all GPS tracking products, there is no single tracking technology—different companies market systems with different permutations—and potential users must become aware of the different kinds of regime that the combined hardware and software can create for particular offenders. Nonetheless, three standard operating modes have evolved for GPS tracking technology, notionally tied to level of assessed risk, all of which monitor the offender's movement incessantly, although only in the first are offenders constantly observed by monitoring staff:

- *Active mode* (for higher risk offenders). This provides a continuous flow of data points in real time using cellular technology. This is both technologically more expensive and requires constant watching by officials. Costs may be offset by requiring the offenders to pay toward the daily cost of the equipment. The offenders can be watched wherever they go or only in relation to the boundaries of one or more exclusion zones they have been told they cannot enter after having been given maps showing clearly where the street boundaries are.
- *Passive mode* (for lower risk offenders). The GPS Unit records location (data points) throughout the day and uploads via landline of cellular means when the offender returns home, probably under curfew, at the end of the day. Supervising officials typically do not read the data until the day afterward. This method can still be used in conjunction with exclusion zones, although not if there is any urgency about keeping offenders out of them. The offenders can be warned not to enter them, and if the uploaded tracking records subsequently show that they did, they will be in violation of their supervision requirements and will be warned or prosecuted accordingly.
- *Hybrid mode*. GPS remains in passive mode or uploads data points at preset intervals unless the offenders violates the rules they are subject to, such as going to the perimeter of an exclusion zone, in which case the active mode kicks in, alerts are sent to monitoring officials and to offenders, and movement is now monitored in real time. Efforts may be made to contact offenders by cell phone, the police may be sent in pursuit of them, and any victims in the exclusion zone may be warned of their possible presence.

Most of the current GPS products are "two piece units" incorporating a waist-worn tracking unit linked (by radio frequency signals) to a conventional ankle bracelet, but four "one piece units" (combining all of the kit in an ankle bracelet) are already on the market, with more promised. The battery in waist-worn units may need recharging in a docking unit installed in the offender's home, requiring return there each night. The rubber/plastic bracelets can be removed, and the tracking unit is not unbreakable but they are fitted with sophisticated (and often patent protected) "anti-tamper devices," commonly based on electrical circuits or optical fibers, although some include "body proximity detectors" (based on temperature) or "motion detectors" (the protracted stillness of the transmitter may indicate that it has been removed or that the wearer is dead). These register "alerts" in the monitoring centers whenever an attempt is made to remove or damage a strap or to open the transmitter itself.

Almost from the start, GPS tracking technology has permitted one-way communication with the offender, using audible or visual signals or vibration that can automatically indicate "battery low" or that the supervising officer should be called or that warns the offender that he or she is nearing an exclusion zone. Most sound alerts are audible only to the offender, but SecureAlert's equipment incorporates a "very loud" siren "designed to draw attention to the client [and that] can be used as punishment or negative reinforcement" (*The Journal of Offender Monitoring*, 2009, p. 68), although it is unclear whether this has ever been used in practice. Some equipment allows two-way communication, permitting the offender to acknowledge receipt of alerts by pager or text (although it makes the kit more costly and harder to miniaturize). At the very least, "alerts and alert acknowledgement reinforce the client's awareness that he or she is under surveillance," but increasingly "more and more agencies are requiring two-way voice communications"—in essence the inclusion of a mobile phone in the kit—enabling the monitoring officers and/or probation officers to engage in periodic dialogue with the mobile offender. It allows officers to interact with their clients about their clients' behavior on a real-time basis" (*The Journal of Offender Monitoring*, 2009, p. 68). While ostensibly adding a "social work"/counseling dimension to the tracking process, there may be a downside to two-way communication; supervisors who are in live contact with offenders who breach an exclusion zone perimeter and still fail to dissuade them from their assumed course of action may incur greater liability for any subsequent crime in the exclusion zone than they would have done if they had merely registered the potential transgression and primed the police to intercept the offenders.

Satellite tracking, like electronic monitoring more generally, makes possible "economies of presence" (Mitchell, 1999) in the offender supervision field. "Economies of presence"—balancing and blending the levels of physical co-presence and remote contact necessary to the accomplishment of a particular social task on the basis of a cost-benefit analysis or a risk assessment—originated in the commercial world and can clearly be applied to "offender supervision." The periodic physical co-presence of probation officer and supervisee in the same building (office or home) was once integral to the very meaning of "supervision"; it was via their structured personal encounters (and sometimes through the relationship that grew between them) that an impact on behavior was effected. Although remote monitoring technologies do not create swathes of "panoptic (viewable) space" in the way that closed-circuit television technologies do, their ability to pinpoint individuals in vast "zones of indistinction" (Agamben, 1997), whether crowded or empty, do enlarge the spatial range over which specific supervisory influence can be exerted over offenders (in "real time"). Nor need they be used in isolation: like house arrest/curfew tagging, GPS tracking potentially adds a surveillant means of gaining compliance to the incentive-based, trust-based, and threat-based means of gaining compliance that have traditionally comprised the social work/correctional repertoire (Nellis, 2007).

Even more important, however, remote monitoring technologies have extended the temporal range of supervision within a given 24-hour period. In the past, the most intensive forms of personalized, humanistic supervision have rarely been more than intermittent, daytime encounters, while curfew tagging only added in an element of control over nighttime activities. Both approaches leave offenders with significant periods of time when they are without the oversight of supervisors, when their whereabouts are unknown or uncertain. It is the temporality of satellite tracking that most distinguishes it from humanistic and relational forms of offender supervision, because it seemingly makes possible incessant oversight—around the clock knowledge of an offender's location in real time or (more usually) some approximation to it—that no personal supervisor could manage and that no traditionally oriented, labor intensive, social work, law enforcement, or correctional agency could afford.

MONITOR AND MONITORED: CONTRASTING EXPERIENCES OF TIME

The monitoring officers watching the computer screens and the individual offender being tracked may be connected in "real time," but there is an asymmetry in the way they experience that "shared" moment. To a degree, on a daily basis, monitoring staff are mentally immersed in distant worlds, albeit worlds that are represented by on-screen or printed-out maps, zones, and schedules with which an offender must abide. Their "now" is not the immediate "here and now" of the office they are sitting in but the simultaneous "now" of events, mostly very mundane events, that are taking place elsewhere. They do not literally see the offender as a physical entity, not even as a visual representation of a physical entity as in a closed-circuit television control center, but rather as a moving dot or arrow leaving electronic trails on "virtual" streets and roads. Two-way text or telephone conversations with the offender may, depending on whether the monitoring officer knows him or her personally, add a sense of the offender's personhood, but in the main the monitoring staff are dealing with "data doubles," simulacra who are defined and judged on the narrow dimension of their spatial behavior and about whom little else may be known. Quite how the experience of temporal proximity to distant people about whom one knows little (but whom one might be imagining as dangerous predators) registers in the minds of the monitors is unknown. One possibility is boredom, and to offset this the process of extended screen watching could be—and is in part already —automated, triggering the monitor's personal attention only when an "incident" occurs, such as a perimeter violation.

What do offenders experience? While subject to GPS tracking offenders are incessantly monitored: every few meters they walk or drive, every place they go, is scanned by a satellite 11,000 miles above them and relayed to a monitoring center. The official assumption is that this will deter them from criminal activity and/or link them to a crime scene if they were present at it. In that sense, their reflexive awareness that "authorities"—local probation or police officers whom they may know or anonymous people in a monitoring center hundreds of miles away—can pinpoint their whereabouts at least creates the possibility of stifling the prospects of them committing a crime, even if tempted, because of the reduced prospects of evading capture. Whether offenders do have a "paranoid" sense of being incessantly monitored, or whether in the course of their daily routines they block it out (perhaps as a defense mechanism, to sustain sanity) is ultimately an empirical question. What is already known is that immediate situational pressures (and their attendant emotions such as frustration and despair) may easily override one's rational awareness of being watched from a distance and precipitate criminal action, and in this sense remote location monitoring is by no means total control, not comprehensively "telematic."

The experience of being tracked is not, however, a wholly passive one; current EM technologies in the United States and Europe remain, in the jargon of the manufacturers, "participant dependent." This term denotes the extent to which offenders must actively comply with the technology if it is to fulfill its locatability function. Compliance always remains a choice. Offenders must resist temptation to cut and discard the bracelet, remember (with two piece, wearable units) to carry the kit with them when they go outdoors, and take responsibility for recharging the battery. The experience of being tracked exemplifies what Adam Crawford (2003) has called "regulated self-regulation" rather than simply being an experience of externally imposed control (see also Paterson, 2007b). In relation to exclusion zones, offenders may experience heightened spatial awareness, even anxiety, lest their actions in a given locality, such as traveling across a corner of their exclusion zone because it is where a particular bus route happens to go or detours one morning, are misinterpreted as transgression by the distant monitors.

While the technology to which offenders are subject may have "killed" distance between them and their monitors, their immediate physical space, the locality in which they live, still matters in a way that is less true for the monitors. The offenders still live in a coterminous "here" and "now," they are embedded in a definite physical locality, and their minds need not routinely be focused elsewhere. For them, the exigencies of everyday life may well be sufficiently absorbing to suppress a constant and vivid sense of electronic connectedness or of exposure to the eyes and minds of others. Their unreflective inattentiveness to this can't ever be total, of course: the kit weighs lightly on the body and needs frequent recharging, prohibited zones and required schedules must be taken into account, and phone calls and texts may be received, but this does not amount to full immersion in "network time." Conversely, for the monitors, attentiveness toward distant offenders will routinely be at the forefront of their minds because this is what they are paid to do. For at least some of their working hours they are immersed in "network time." They know precisely where distant people are, even if they are not "virtually" interacting with them. Without access to other forms of intelligence, or of communication with them, they cannot know more than their location, and if they infer from this or their pattern of movement that a crime could be, is being, or has been committed, their capacity to intervene in real time is negligible. This may not remain so, but understanding what the future may hold in this field requires a detour into the once imagined past of offender tracking.

THE (IMAGINED PAST) FUTURES OF OFFENDER TRACKING

I will begin this exploration by drawing on the work of Paul Virilio (1997, 2006). There are, it has to be admitted, certain risks in doing this, because unlike Castells's, Virilio's analysis is an unashamedly normative, almost apocalyptic portrayal of the impact of "speed machines" and "vision machines" on contemporary life. He recognizes two temporal orders: the "good" natural order of rootedness, sequence, and rhythm, and the "bad," disembedded order of simultaneous electronic communication, often writing as if the latter had already eclipsed the former, to the manifest detriment of attentiveness to our immediate physical and social space and the "flesh and blood" people in it. Extensive immersion in real-time encounters with distant others, he fears, will produce a diminished sociality in the "here and now"; interaction between people who are merely digital/"spectral" presences to one another will fray the bonds of an already tenuous sense of common humanity.

Nonetheless, despite this bleak prejudgment, Virilio must at least be credited with foreseeing some of the issues that real-time communication might raise, and he is perhaps best understood as challenging the "over-hyped remote telepresence" that is undoubtedly idealized by the telecommunication industry, particularly in advertisements for, say, mobile phones and social networking sites, or (as we have already seen) for GPS satellite tracking. One of Virilio's key speculations about "optoelectronics" is that it will inexorably evolve from merely watching at a distance to acting (or affecting the behavior of the watched) at a distance, a movement from the "permanent telesurveillance" of the masses towards the "widespread remote control" of individuals, or "tactile telepresence." The bases of this belief were the already emerging technologies of telemedicine and smart homes (Virilio, 1997, p. 14), in which wearable or body-implanted devices or sensors in one's immediate environment would remotely monitor the life signs of the old, the disabled, and the demented. Telemedicine may well be part of our medical futures (and may not be perceived in the sinister way that Virilio perceives it), but whether it is a template for, or a precursor of, other and more ubiquitous forms of "tactile telepresence" is a far more debatable point.

Had Virilio known of the satellite tracking of offenders, his worst fears about its likely trajectory would doubtless have been confirmed by the knowledge that the capacity to "zap" tracked offenders had already been inscribed as an imaginative and desirable possibility in the prehistory of these technologies. The Schwitzgebel brothers who pioneered what we now call "electronic monitoring" did adapt guided missile technology to track offenders in Boston in the late 1960s and early 1970s but did no more than use tonal communication and "walkie talkies" to affect the behavior of their experimental subjects (and were committed to using EM as rehabilitation, not punitively) (Schwitzgebel, 1964: Gable & Gable, 2005). Some of their contemporaries in the field dreamed far darker dreams. Computer scientist Joseph Meyer (1971) considered as feasible, even then, a terrestrial "transponder [not a satellite-based] surveillance system" in which a nationwide network of computer-linked transceivers, high on the walls of buildings (outside and in) in every neighborhood, would pick up in real time a unique radio-frequency identifier signal from unremovable "transponders" attached to the wrists of some 25 million convicted criminals (usually released from prison) in the United States. Curfew and territorial restrictions could be programmed into the system, tailored to individual offenders, and some transceivers would cause any nearby transponder to sound an alarm, warning the wearer to keep away and (probably) drawing attention to him or her. Criminologists Ingraham and Smith (1972), influenced by recent research on the "electrical stimulation of the brain" (ESB), envisaged and desired something much more intrusive:

> In the very near future, a computer technology will make possible alternatives to imprisonment. The development of systems for telemetering information from sensors implanted in or on the body will soon make

possible the observation and control of human behavior without actual physical contact. Through such telemetric devices, it will be possible to maintain twenty-four-hour-a-day surveillance over the subject and to intervene electronically or physically to influence and control selected behavior and from a distance without physical contact. The possible implications for criminology and corrections of such telemetric systems is tremendously significant. (p. 35)

Simply because these technologies did not come to pass it is difficult to recall how seriously they were once taken in certain professional circles, how plausible (and to some, fearful) they once seemed. They did understandably arouse political opposition, and this, along with commercial-technical limitations on their development, did help to suppress them (Mitford, 1973; Schrag, 1978). But tracking-and-zapping remained linked in the popular imagination if not necessarily the professional one, and in the Spider-Man story that famously played a (minor) part in the genesis of the first court ordered electronically monitored house arrest in the United States in 1982, the tracking device locked on the superhero's arm (by a villain) had been set to explode if he tried to remove it (Burrell & Gable, 2008). The question of zapping never in fact arose in respect of "first generation" EM house arrest technology, although the development of "remote alcohol monitoring"— periodically checking the alcohol intake of curfewed offenders using a breathalyzer linked to the home-based monitoring device—introduced an element of "tactile telepresence" into the arrangement (which can be replicated, using perspiration monitoring technology in tracking systems). Nonetheless, in the era when mere house arrest began to be seen as a somewhat limited and incomplete use of EM, when the ideal of tracking offender movements over a wide area rather than simply restricting them to a single place resurfaced (because it now seemed technically feasible), the zapping/tracking link arose again. Colorado probation officer Max Winkler's (1991) proposal for electronic "walking prisons" (a concept already explored in a science fiction story by Cynthia Bunn in 1974) included the possibility of being able to "zap" offenders from a distance, although when he became involved with the engineers who first patented tracking technology, the idea was dropped (Hoshen, Sennott, & Winkler, 1995).

GPS has become established in the United States without recourse to zapping, and while some of those involved in it may share Winkler's aspirations, there are doubtless many who are convinced that while tracking per se is ethically acceptable, extending it to remotely inflict physical pain is a punitive step too far. Such people, however, no longer have the luxury of doubting that zapping is technically possible. A tracking device that could remotely administer an electric shock to an offender poised to cross the perimeter of an exclusion zone by fully discharging the battery that powers the ankle-worn transmitter has been created by Shadow Tagging in South Africa

(House, 2009). It has not been used, and it indeed has caused some consternation in the EM industry whose commercial interests in Europe and the United States may be threatened if EM, already prone to unwelcome associations with "Big Brother," became publicly tainted, even conceptually, with pain infliction as well.

It is unlikely that zapping technologies would even be under discussion if offender tracking did not already entail and require a degree of depersonalization. Offenders, especially violent or sexual offenders, are easily depersonalized, rendered less human than the law-abiding, imbued with an unfathomable "otherness" that is in turn used to justify hatred and rejection of the offender, and the subsequent imposition of suffering and stigma. It does not take technology to create or impute this sense of otherness to offenders, but the greater the social distance between supervisor and offender and the less humanly rounded the offender can be made to seem, the less need (and the less possibility) there is for empathy. Tracking technology can aggravate this tendency. To be reduced to a moving dot on a screen map, to be watched as a mere simulation is not, as a therapist might put it, "to be met as a person" (McCluskey, 2005). Remote location monitoring involves an even more attenuated sense of telepresence than the visual surveillance entailed by closed-circuit television, which at least "depicts" recognizable people. In Virilio's somewhat grandiose terms, remote location monitoring entails "a transmutation in the 'depth of field' and so in the optical density of the human environment" (Virilio, 1997, p. 24) that reduces people to the most minimal of "data doubles," the most meager analogues of their real selves. The in-built depersonalizing features of tracking technology may well be muted or neutralized, even reversed, in situations where the monitors, be they probation or police officers, have personal, proximity-based knowledge of the offender concerned. Proximity, however, never guarantees that a stigmatized and objectified individual will be treated with humanity, and some professionals may well find it easier to be cordial toward offenders when they are nothing more than remote, disembodied digital presences.

While there is no reason to assume that current versions of offender tracking will *necessarily* segue into more punitive versions, it is not too difficult to understand where the lure and logic of the idea comes from. Real-time tracking can create a situation in which remote monitors may well believe that an offender is about to enter an exclusion zone but may not be in a position to prevent it. Texting or phoning the offender, if the equipment permits this, may not be sufficient. At such moments the brute facts of geography— the distance of the offender from the monitor—reassert themselves, because meaningful intervention requires police "on the ground" to get to wherever the offender is before any harm is done, and there may not be sufficient time to do this. In such circumstances, to assuage the monitor's sense of helplessness and protect a potential victim, the emotional and practical appeal of remote intervention can readily be appreciated, especially as it is backed up, culturally, with a raft of science fiction stories that often put a positive spin on such devices and, more dramatically still, by the contemporary reality of unmanned aerial vehicles ("drones") piloted from an air force base in Nevada being used to assassinate "the enemy" in Iraq, Pakistan, and Afghanistan (Singer, 2009). Will the risks of perimeter-crossing ever be deemed so great that remote pain infliction comes to seem necessary? In the United States, the question may one day be posed. More immediately, speculative anxiety about the "putatively worse" scenario of zapping actually deflects attention from what is already problematic and alarming about actually existing GPS tracking. Even without zapping, the prospect of subjecting thousands of offenders to incessant oversight without well-reasoned justification remains a chilling one.

CONCLUSION: THE PROSPECT OF ETERNAL VIGILANCE

It was once said, in the preelectronic age, that the price of freedom is eternal vigilance, that good men must forever be on the alert for incipient tyranny if democracy was to be preserved. In our emergent, high-tech "surveillance societies," the very real possibility of a once unimaginable form of "eternal vigilance" is coming to be seen as a threat to individual freedom rather than the guarantor of it. In the United States, public unease about this prospect was brought into sharp focus by the controversy surrounding the post 9/11 proposal for a "total information awareness" strategy, and while it never came to pass in the form envisaged, a significant expansion of data collection on American citizens has nonetheless been its legacy (Whitaker, 2006). These developments have been imagined and conceptualized (and anticipated) by a number of writers using different terms and phrases, sometimes veering to the hyperbolic; for example, the "superpanopticon" (Poster, 1990), "the maximum surveillance society" (Marx, 1988), and "hypercontrol" (Bogard, 1996). James Rule's (2002) concept of "perpetual contact" neatly captures the tangible temporal reality in which these imaginaries are grounded. Depending on the political and professional decisions that are made about its use, satellite tracking can, by exploiting the already existing capacity for "relentless connectivity" (Castells et al., 2006, p. 248), make possible "incessant oversight" or what I have here called (also hyperbolically) "eternal vigilance." It is one aspect among many of a burgeoning "surveillant assemblage" (Haggerty & Ericson, 2000) targeted specifically at offenders whose monitored locations and schedules become loosely analogous to the regimented space of the prison.

The released sex offenders who, in the legislation of over 20 American states, may in the future be placed on satellite tracking for the remainder of their lives, whose locations will be immediately knowable under active regimes, whose movements, even under passive regimes, will be inscribed moment by moment in searchable databases, making them forever traceable, will to all intents and purposes be subject to the eternal vigilance of the authorities. While on parole, they may at least be involved in programs that seek to challenge and change their behavior, but once the parole period has ended, only tracking remains, the shared responsibility of law enforcement officials and GPS monitoring organizations rather than correctional officers (International Association of Chiefs of Police 2009). Notwithstanding the dangers that such sex offenders pose, the admitted difficulties of managing them, and the high levels of communal fear that they arouse, there is, as Button, DeMichele, and Payne (2009) point out, no clear rationale for lifelong tracking, no undisputed connection between typical patterns of recidivism and a need for incessant oversight other than the simple capacity to trace all past movements, which may deter as well as aid detection. In addition, offenders may prefer tracking to incarceration, but is any of this justification enough? All American citizens are under greater surveillance and are more locatable than hitherto (with greater and lesser degrees of awareness and anxiety about it) and may have only limited concerns about those transgressors among them who are subject to even more intensive forms of locatability. Nonetheless the prospective consequences for citizenship of having a cohort of the population, however small, however stigmatized, subject to the eternal vigilance of law enforcement and commercial agencies—quite apart from its impact on the subjectivities of those concerned—warrants the preliminary moral scrutiny of satellite tracking that has been offered here and invites further work on the nature of the control that it entails.

REFERENCES

Adam, B. (2004). *Time.* Cambridge, UK: Polity Press.

Agamben, G. (1997). *Homo sacer: Sovereign power and bare life.* Stanford, CA: Stanford University Press.

Bauman, Z. (2000). *Liquid modernity.* Cambridge: Polity Press.

Benshoof, P. (2007). Over-reliance on any technology would leave us vulnerable. *Border and Transportation Security,* 147–148. (www.gdsinternational.com/infocentre)

Bogard, W. (1996). *The simulation of surveillance: Hypercontrol in telematic societies.* Cambridge: Cambridge University Press.

Bogard, W. (2006). Welcome to the society of control: The simulation of surveillance revisited. In K. D. Haggerty & R. V. Ericson (Eds.), *Surveillance and visibility.* Toronto: University of Toronto Press.

Buck, J. (2009). *The basics: GPS tracking in community corrections.* Boulder, CO: BI Incorporated.

Bunn, C. (1974). And keep us from our castles. In J. D. Olander & M. H. Greenberg (Eds.), (1977). *Criminal justice through science fiction* (pp. 168–194). New York: New Viewpoints.

Burrell, W., & Gable, R. (2008). From B. F. Skinner to Spiderman to Martha Stewart: The past, present and future of electronic monitoring of offenders. *Journal of Offender Rehabilitation, 46*(3&4), 101–118.

Burroughs, W. (1986). *The adding machine: Collected essays.* New York: Seaver Books.

Button, D. M., DeMichele, M., & Payne, B. K. (2009). Using electronic monitoring to supervise sex offenders: Legislative patterns and implications for community corrections officers. *Criminal Justice Policy Review, 20,* 1–23.

Castells, M. (1996). *The rise of the network society,* (2nd ed.). Oxford: Blackwell.

Castells, M., Fernandez-Ardevol, M., Qiu, J. L., & Aey, A. (2006). *Mobile communications and society: A global perspective.* Cambridge, MA: MIT Press.

Christie, N. (2000). *Crime control as industry.* London: Routledge.

Crawford, A. (2003). Contractual governance of deviant behavior. *Journal of Law and Society, 30*(4), 479–505.

Doffing, D. (2010). Is there a future for RF in a GPS world? *Journal of Offender Monitoring, 22*(1), 12–15.

Elzinga, H., & Nijboer, J. A. (2006). Probation supervision using GPS. *European Journal of Crime, Criminal Law and Criminal Justice, 14*(4), 366–381.

Gable, R. S., & Gable, R. K. (2005). Increasing the effectiveness of electronic monitoring. *Perspectives: The Journal of the American Probation and Parole Association, 31*(1), 24–29.

Genosko, G., & Thompson, S. (2006). Tense theory: The temporalities of surveillance. In D. Lyon (Ed.), *Theorising surveillance: The panopticon and beyond.* Cullompton: Willan.

Haggerty, K. D., & Ericson, R. V. (2000). The surveillant assemblage. *British Journal of Sociology, 51,* 605–622.

Haggerty, K. D., & Ericson, R. V. (2001). The military technostructures of policing. In P. B. Kraska (Ed.), *Militarising the American criminal justice system.* Boston: Northeastern University Press.

Hoshen, J., Sennott, J., & Winkler, M. (1995). Keeping tabs on criminals. *Spectrum IEEE, 32*(2), 26–32.

House, D. (2009). Shadow tagging systems. Paper presented at the Conference Permanente Europeene de la Probation, May 7–9.

Ingraham, B. L., & Smith, G. S. (1972). The use of electronics in the observation and control of human behavior and its possible use in rehabilitation and parole. *Issues in Criminology, 7*(2).

International Association of Chiefs of Police. (2008). *Tracking sex offenders with electronic monitoring technology: Implications and practical uses for law enforcement.* Washington, DC: International Association of Chiefs of Police.

Journal of Offender Monitoring, 20(1–2). (2009). Special issue on the 2008–2009 Electronic Monitoring Survey.

Lilly, J. R. (1992). Selling justice: Electronic monitoring and the security industry. *Justice Quarterly, 9,* 493–503.

Lilly, J. R., & Deflem, M. (1996). Profit and penality: An analysis of the corrections-commercial complex. *Crime and Delinquency, 42*, 3–20.

Lilly, J. R., & Knepper, P. (1993). An international perspective on the privatisation of corrections. *Howard Journal, 31*, 174–191.

Lyon, D. (2006). Why where you are matters: mundane mobilities, transparent technologies and digital discrimination. In T. Monahan (Ed.), *Surveillance and security: Technological politics and everyday life*. London: Routledge.

Marx, G. (1988). *Undercover: Police surveillance in America*. Berkeley: University of California Press.

McLuskey, U. (2005). *To be met as a person: The dynamics of attachment in professional encounters*. London: Karnac.

Meyer, J. A. (1970). Crime deterrent transponder system. *IEEE Transactions on Aerospace and Electronic Systems*, Vol *AES-7*(1), 2–22.

Mitchell, W. (1999). *E-topia: Urban life, Jim, but not as we know it*. Cambridge: The MIT Press.

Mitford, J. (1973). *Kind and unusual punishment; The prison business*. New York: Knopf.

Monmonier, M. (2004). *Spying with maps: Surveillance technologies and the future of privacy*. Chicago: University of Chicago Press.

Moore, M., & Thurston, J. (2009). *County correctional issues: Adapting in an era of jail overcrowding, tight budgets, rising costs and changing inmate demographies. White paper*. Boulder, CO: BI Incorporated.

Nellis, M. (2006). Electronic monitoring, satellite tracking and the new punitiveness in England and Wales. In J. Pratt, D. Brown, M. Brown, S. Hallsworth, & W. Morrison (Eds.), *The new punitiveness: Trends, theories and perspectives*. Cullompton: Willan.

Nellis, M. (2007). Surveillance, rehabilitation and electronic monitoring: Getting the issues clear. *Criminology and Public Policy, 5*(1), 103–108.

Nellis, M. (2009a). 24/7/365. Mobility, locatability and the satellite tracking of offenders. In A. K. Franco, H. O. Gundus, & H. M. Lommell (Eds.), *Technologies of insecurity: The surveilance of everyday life*. London: Routledge.

Nellis, M. (2009b). Electronic monitoring and penal control in a telematic society. In J. Doakes, P. Knepper, & J. Shapland (Eds.), *Urban crime prevention, surveillance and restorative justice: Effects of social technologies*. Boca Raton, FL: CRC Press.

Paterson, C. (2007a). Commercial crime control and the electronic monitoring of offenders. *Social Justice, 34*(3–4), 98–110.

Paterson, C. (2007b). Street-level surveillance: Human agency and the electronic monitoring of offenders. *Surveillance and Society, 4*(4), 314–328.

Poster, M. (1990). *The mode of information: Postmodernism and social context*. Chicago: University of Chicago Press.

Rule, J. (2002). From mass society to perpetual contact. In J. E. Katz & Aakhus (Eds.), *Perpetual contact: Mobile communication, privacy talk, public performance*. Cambridge: Cambridge University Press.

Schrag, P. (1978). *Mind control*. New York: Dell Publishing.

Schwitzgebel, R. (1964). *Streetcorner research: An experimental approach to the juvenile delinquent*. Cambridge, MA: Harvard University Press.

Shute, S. (2007). *Satellite tracking of offenders: A study of the pilots in England and wales* (Research summary 4). London: Ministry of Justice.

Singer, P. (2009). *Wired for war: The robotics revolution and conflict in the 21st century*. London: Penguin.

Stacey, T. (1995). Innovations in technology. In K. Schulz (Ed.), *Electronic monitoring and corrections: The policy, the operation, the research*. Vancouver: Simon Fraser University.

Tomlinson, J. (2007). *The culture of speed: The coming of immediacy*. London Sage.

Virilio, P. (1997). *Open sky*. London: Verso.

Virilio, P. (2006). *Speed and politics*. Los Angeles: Semiotext(e).

Whitaker, R. (2006, July–August). A Faustian bargain? American and the dream of total information awareness. In K. D. Haggerty & R. V. Erickson (Eds.), *The new politics of surveillance and visibility*. Toronto: University of Toronto Press.

Winkler, M. (1991). Walking prisons: The developing technology of electronic controls. *The Futurist*, 34–36.

Ethical Considerations Around the Implementation of Telecare Technologies

ANDREW ECCLES

Glasgow School of Social Work, a Joint School of Glasgow and Strathclyde Universities

The use of assistive technology in social care, through a program of telecare, has become a prominent feature of policy development in some advanced industrial societies. This article looks at developments in Scotland, where ambitious targets for the application of telecare technologies are underway. The focus here is on telecare for older people. The paper starts by examining the discourse around demographic change and fiscal pressures to explore an increased use of technology. The paper then examines ethical issues raised by this telecare program and argues that the frameworks in use, while important, are limited in scope. It thus considers wider ethical frames of reference and looks at policy imperatives—such as interprofessional working and a performance driven culture—that may make ethical considerations more difficult to realize in practice.

INTRODUCTION

The use of assistive technology (AT) has attained greater prominence in the delivery of health and social care in recent years and is set to expand more significantly in the near future. This paper looks at the use of assistive technologies in social care—its telecare format—and considers a number of issues that might have ethical impact in the course of implementation. Three areas are broached: first, the policy discourse that has grown up around the implementation of telecare; second, some of the ethical issues arising from the use of such technology and ethical codes that accompany its use; and, third, the evaluation of the effectiveness of the technology. The paper takes a case study approach with reference to the current situation in Scotland. The focus is primarily on telecare policy for older people, by some measure the area of most usage and financial commitment by government. The approach here is to review policy implementation in light of published documents and policy evaluation. The paper starts with some comment on the policy context for telecare and a survey of current policy intentions.

Policy Context

Scotland has a population of some five million people, unevenly spread across a geographical landscape that has alternatively a dense lowland population (the central belt) and a more dispersed population in less easily accessible terrain. In common with most other advanced industrial societies, the population is projected to have a greater 65 plus age element in future (with particularly high growth in the number of citizens aged 75 and over). Equally, Scotland has had a declining birth rate over the past 20 years (General Register Office for Scotland, 2009). It is also a devolved polity, with different (and more costly) arrangements from the rest of the United Kingdom (UK) for its health and social care. As immigration policy remains part of a UK policy remit, ways of addressing this demographic change (for example, an immigrant care workforce) are limited. In keeping with most advanced industrial societies discussion about older people among policymakers quickly turns to the question of how best to meet future health and social care needs and their attendant costs (Lymbery, 2005).

Since 2006 Scotland has embarked on an ambitious program of employing technological solutions to care needs under the auspices of the then Scottish Executive's telecare development program. Telecare is defined by the program as a generic term for a range of technologies used in "the continuous, automatic and remote monitoring of care needs" (Scottish Government, 2008b). Specific targets for its deployment were laid out in the document *Seizing the Opportunity: Telecare Strategy 2008–10* (Scottish Government, 2008a). These objectives, for the year 2015, envisage that

> all new homes, public and private, and all refurbished social housing, will be fitted with the capacity for care and health services to be provided interactively via broadband from day one of occupation; telehealth will be widely recognised by service users and their carers as the route to greater independence and quality of life; independent evaluation will confirm that no care service users in Scotland who could benefit from telecare services in a home-based setting remain in an institutional environment; [and] remote long term condition monitoring undertaken from home will be the norm. (p. 6)

Furthermore the program argues that in the process Scotland will be "recognised as an innovative world leader in the provision of care and health services based on telecare technology" (Scottish Government, 2008a, p. 6). The primary objectives of this ambitious program are sixfold: reduce the number of avoidable emergency admissions and readmissions to hospital, increase the speed of discharge from hospital once clinical need is met, reduce the use of care homes, improve the quality of life of users of telecare services, reduce the pressure on (informal) carers, and support effective procurement to ensure that telecare services grow as quickly as possible. Underpinning this is a clear commitment to "achieve efficiencies (cash releasing or time releasing)" (Scottish Government, 2009, p. 3).

There is a growing literature offering evidence of the benefits of the use of assistive technology with older people (Scottish Government, 2009; Loader, Hardey, & Keeble, 2009; McCreadie & Tinker, 2005). These benefits include an increase in independence for service users, reassurance for carers and family members, and the potential to release costs from social care budgets for alternative provision. This paper takes no issue with the research on the potential for advantage afforded by this technology. It does argue, however, that some areas of current policy implementation warrant scrutiny. These areas include the limited policy discussion of alternative models of care, the limited ethical frameworks currently in use, and performance measurement criteria that may encourage less than optimal practice.

Policy Discourse

The policy discourse emerging around telecare policy and older people centers explicitly on dealing with patterns of demographic change and the "old-age dependency ratio" (European Union Public Health Information System, 2009) between older people and a working population. There are dangers, in that this terminology may suggest older people will axiomatically become dependant. Tinker (1997) offers a measured take on the dependency thesis and how patterns of the ratio have changed over the decades. Nonetheless, a persuasive discourse about the imperative for new ways of delivering care to deal with the dependency ratio has fast emerged. Sometimes the language here is noticeably less measured; for example, Tunstall, the recognized telecare technology delivery partner of the Scottish Government, argues that the United Kingdom "is sitting on a demographic time bomb" (Tunstall, 2009, p. 3). These demographic changes are indeed formidable, but the evidence around population change is complex. Older people's own assessment of their health is consistently more optimistic than that of expert medical opinion, so there may be different constructions of care requirements here (Bowling & Dieppe, 2005), while the whole territory of the social construction of old age (Townsend, 2006) presents itself at the center of these arguments. Thus, whether through the rubric of policy objectives or the management of performance indicators, a powerful discourse has emerged about technology as a solution to the perceived scale of the fiscal challenges presented by demographic change. This is not to discount the potential gains—particularly independent living—for service users, but the financing of care needs frames much of the debate among policymakers.

There emerges something of a conflation between the merits of technology and fiscal efficiency here. In the absence of a sound methodology to examine the impact of technology on costs and a longitudinal study of the impact of technology on people's quality of life, why should it be supposed that telecare use "grow as quickly as possible" (Scottish Government, 2009, p. 4) or that "Telecare and Telehealth will be widely recognized by service users and their carers as the route to greater independence and quality of life" (Scottish Government, 2008a, p. 6)? These demographic challenges might equally afford space to rethink our understanding of care needs and reconfigure the way in which communities might address these needs (see Freedland [2009] for an overview of this debate). An alternative approach might also serve to reappraise a social policy system increasingly driven by an agenda of linking welfare provision to work (Page, 2007) in recent years.

In this vein, Mort, Roberts, and Milligan (2009) argue that there is a need to address an "ethical and democratic deficit in this field which has arisen due to a proliferation in research and development of advanced care technologies that has not been accompanied by sufficient consideration of their social context" (p. 85). As it stands, policy appears to be driven by technological possibilities that are underpinned by an assumed fiscal imperative in the face of demographic change. The demographics are indeed stark and technological solutions here clearly have utility and will continue to confer benefit. But technology continues to be also rather seductive to bureaucrats and policymakers as a way of addressing complex social change despite past evidence of failure and expense (see, for example, Taylor, Groleau, Heaton, & Van Every, 2000).

ETHICAL FRAMEWORKS IN TELECARE

The ethical frameworks currently employed by the various agencies engaged in the provision of telecare are limited in scope and unevenly interpreted. These limits in scope are grounded in practical reality: ethical frameworks have to be understood by practitioners, and their terminology has to resonate with care assessment. Reviewing the discussion across various telecare forums, it is clear that ethical considerations play a relatively minor role amid wider discussion of client groups, service delivery, and technological potential. The key ethical frameworks in use are essentially biomedical and best summarized around four principles that have long been the mainstay of biomedical enquiry. They are discussed to good effect by Beauchamp and Childress (2001) in their classic text *Biomedical Ethics* and have been adopted across both health and social care, such as by the ASTRID project on dementia care (Frisby, 2000).

The principles embrace autonomy, beneficence, nonmalfeasance, and justice. These are powerful and important concepts. They are also limited in their scope, historically shaped, and unevenly relevant across different cultural settings. Moreover, much of the discussion in biomedical ethics centers on more acute treatment, invasive procedures, and end of life decision making, which are not features that register prominently in considerations around social care. Even then, within the context of telecare, these concepts are differently interpreted across different agencies. For example, in the United Kingdom context, the Care Services Improvement Partnership (CSIP) argues that an understanding of beneficence "involves finding the balance between risk tolerance and risk aversion. There may be a dilemma between beneficence and safety & independence" (Care Services Improvement Partnership, 2005, p. 2), while the Scottish government notes in its summary on ethical issues, drawing on the ASTRID framework, "we should try to do good to the people we care for" (Scottish Government, 2007, n.p.). Nonmalfeasance, the CSIP advises, "will involve a balance between avoiding harm and respecting decisions about dignity, integrity and preferences" (Care Services Improvement Partnership, 2005, p. 2), while the Scottish government guidance notes that "we should try to avoid doing people harm" (Scottish Government, 2007, n.p.). These are quite different understandings of key ethical issues that may translate into different approaches in practice settings.

The primacy of autonomy (Wilmot, 1997) in community care policy sits at the heart of much of the telecare agenda. This importance placed on autonomy arguably underplays the significance of the interdependence of human affairs (Wilmot, 1997; Barnes, 2006), and unpacking arguments around autonomy in any development in community care is rarely straightforward. This would be particularly the case across different cultural settings, where interdependence may be more highly prized and notions of need quite differently understood (Tao & Drover, 1997), which raises further questions about the utility of the biomedical framework in complex multicultural community settings. While the objective of reductions in residential care home admissions in the telecare agenda may often be laudable, a cursory look at the history of the development of community care in United Kingdom over the past 20 years suggests that a primary driver in the move from institutional care to "care in the community" has been fiscal (Morbey, Smith, & Means, 2002; Means, Richards, & Smith, 2008).

There is evidence that the use of technology can alleviate isolation among older people (Blaschke, Freddolino, & Mullen, 2009). But the picture here is complex and demands further research. The ASTRID framework mentioned previously notes that increased autonomy, in its guise of greater independence, might bring with it isolation among service users, in line with Wilmot's notion of "unwanted autonomy" (Wilmot, 1997), while Lowe (2009) discusses the potential for telecare technology to increase isolation and the subsequent link between isolation and clinical depression. Thus, one factor in any method of calculating cost savings through the use of technology might want to include potential attendant costs for health care if depression were to increase. Additional considerations here would be the quality of care that any such increase in depression through isolation might engender, its potential for not being diagnosed and, even if detected, how adequately it might be dealt with in the health care system. Current telecare policy in Scotland recognizes this potential for isolation in the call for the development of a system of "befrienders" to provide human contact, to be developed in tandem as the use of telecare increases (Scottish Government, 2008). But this is an area that is adversely affected by the fiscal pressures in local care services and the voluntary sector. Thus one of the ironies of the increased use of technology to tackle care home admissions might be a form of increased institutionalization, through isolation, within recipients' own homes.

Again, the picture here is complex, as evidence cuts both ways; there is a need for an understanding of how technology might decrease isolation for some people through greater connectedness but potentially increase it for others through reluctance to engage with the technological potential or from an absence of human contact. The key element here is an understanding of the social context in which technology is being applied. The moot point is whether this sits consistently with the policy aim for rapid growth in the use of telecare. Given that this *is* the current policy objective, the debate on the use of telecare technologies will be taking place within a situation of existing and rapid deployment.

Differences in interpretation among agencies advising on telecare provision around issues of beneficence and nonmalfeasance have been noted previously. Even if there were greater consistency of interpretation, decision making would, in any case, be contextual. If there was a risk of increased isolation through the use of technology this was offset by the wish of telecare recipients to remain in their own homes, and some risk/benefit calculus could be employed, but more evidence on how these decisions are in fact calculated across different implementing agencies is needed, as "doing good" and "avoiding harm" are invariably actions grounded in complex social situations. Two questions emerge here: is a biomedical ethical framework adequate for the needs of different telecare user groups, and are assessments of the need for assistive technologies sensitive enough (for example, in assessing risk) in the interpretation of this framework? If the policy objective remains a "rapid expansion" of the use of telecare, but particular constituencies (across age groups or geographical location) have different attitudes to its use, how is sensitivity to this to be realized, particularly when performance targets are partly based on technology budget spend?

Besides autonomy, beneficence, and nonmalfeasance, Beauchamp and Childress (2001) include justice in their key principles. This is picked up by implementing agencies. On this the Scottish government (2007) concludes, "People should be treated fairly and equally." There is scope in this statement to discuss how this fairness and equity might be demonstrated. In a clinical setting this might involve two patients receiving the same treatment for the same condition (although in reality this decision would be tempered by quality of life years and perhaps also current lifestyles). In a wider social context there exists a parallel government policy agenda committed to the pursuit of social justice. In this case there may be a sound argument for *unequal* treatment to address social inequality. Be that as it may, there are interesting aspects to any discussion of social justice and technology arising through the fast-moving telecare agenda. Key elements of second generation telecare (monitoring the movement of people in their own homes, for example, prior to deciding on care packages) require at least a telephone landline, while broadband access would offer a clear advantage to allow the families of telecare users to become engaged in this process of monitoring. However, the technology trends in some of the more socially disadvantaged areas of Scotland are uneven: while broadband installation is under way in some social housing, elsewhere the cost of telephone landline installation and service has given way to cheaper alternatives such as "pay as you go" mobile telephones with more limited connectivity (Eccles, 2009). This prospect of a digital divide in social care has been rehearsed more generally (Steyaert & Gould, 2009); here the specifics warrant attention, as the ability to access and negotiate the use of technology underpins the utility of telecare development.

While it is older people who are the main subject of current telecare policy, telecare itself has application across a range of groups of people. It may have a particularly liberating application for people with physical disability where the argument has long been made that traditional care relationships based on human contact are potentially demeaning and oppressive (Barnes, 2006). Thus the implications of increased autonomy might take on a very different complexion between different recipient telecare groups. The point is that, to date, the ethical frameworks predominantly being used serve an important but essentially limited function and are open to different interpretations even in their status as guidelines. That it remains essentially a biomedical framework in application to situations of social care prompts the need for other sources of ethical inquiry. It is not being suggested here that the already complex task of making care decisions should be subject to a further accretion of ethical principles or approaches in dealing directly with telecare users (see Sommerville [2003] for a useful discussion here). Nonetheless, as will be discussed, more socially grounded ethical approaches do exist, and these might usefully inform a broader ethical awareness in discussions around the role of technology in human services.

Additional Ethical Approaches in Telecare

The next section of this paper explores other ethical approaches in relation to the use of telecare technologies that may be worth consideration. There is a burgeoning literature around technology ethics (see Ratto [2007] for an overview). Even as the "four principles" of ethical consideration in common usage do not lend themselves to use in a "checklist" approach (although such procedures have become a more prevalent feature of a managerialist culture in social services in recent years), alternative approaches lend themselves even less to clear-cut application. That managerialism abhors messiness should not, however, preclude their consideration. Equally, alternative approaches are not necessarily concerned with developing new ethical theory around ethics and technology; for example, Johnstone's discussion of ethical approaches that are based on capability theory in computer ethics draws on Aristotle's notion of the flourishing life (Johnstone, 2007). Two approaches, each of which raises useful lines of inquiry about the increased use of telecare technologies, come from the traditions of an ethic of care (Held, 2006; Noddings, 1984; Tronto, 1993) and intuitional ethics (Driver, 2007). Neither features in the ethical frameworks routinely employed in telecare implementation (which tends to embrace the four principles), and certainly neither would lend themselves to straightforward use in assessing, despite their particular relevance to the field of community-based medicine and social care. Their application to the whole question of the use of telecare technology as a strategy is, however, certainly relevant.

AN ETHIC OF CARE

It is precisely in this field of community health and social care that interaction between professions and service users might exist on a relationship developed and sustained over a longer period of time than in acute medical settings that inform the "four principles" outlined previously. Barnes (2006) notes the way in which care workers go beyond tasks to develop relationships over and above contractual obligations, taking the argument into the territory of an "ethic of care," with its emphasis on relational approaches to care that are, above all, contextual and not necessarily uniform in their approach. This enquiry posits care as a *moral* activity based on a complex array of obligations and reciprocities. A simple example of this might be care workers going beyond contractual obligations; for example, spending more time to ensure continuity in care recipients' lives or making additional visits in passing to particular clients with whom the care worker has developed a relationship perhaps over a number of years. Some older people value independence highly and might regard being the recipient of this type of care invasive or demeaning, a sign of a loss of faculty. Others might welcome greater human intervention, particularly if they have lost lifelong partners.

Equally, these patterns will not be fixed over time. This relational aspect to care may thus be played out quite differently in different settings. Recent studies of the use of technology with older people allude to this complexity. Hanson, Osipovic, and Percival (2009), in their evaluation of Lifestyle Monitoring Devices, conclude:

> In order to make "sense of sensors," alongside the data provided by the devices one needs rich contextual information that is normally accumulated through social interactions between caregivers and care receivers, a two-way communication process that can best be described as a "dialogue of care." (p. 111)

On the other hand, Pols and Moser (2009, p. 160) note, "In discussions about the use of new technologies in health care, including the most recent versions appearing as 'telecare,' there is the fear that cold technologies will be implemented at the cost of warm human care"; however they conclude from their research that "the opposition between cold technology and warm care does not hold," but that "there are different relations between people and technologies within different use practices allowing different affective and social relations" (Pols and Moser, 2009, p. 159). The context of relationships is thus crucial.

This relational aspect cuts both ways; care workers themselves may derive satisfaction from their relations with clients (Philips, 2007), and this may prompt an unreasonable reluctance on the part of care workers to engage with technology where the relations that have developed with service users are strong (or indeed where care workers' employment is threatened). If technology is viewed as an imperative in managing the demands thrown up by demographic change, how are relationships and contextual sensitivity to be recognized without more complex ethical frames of reference and enquiry?

INTUITIONISM

Another aspect of the remote delivery of care—for example, through monitoring and surveillance—centers on the qualitative difference to ethical judgements that might result from different types of care. Intuitionism opens up lines for reflection here (Driver, 2007). Intuitive responses to right and wrong courses of action in the face of immediate human dilemmas are less likely to be played out when the ethical dilemmas are more remote or abstract. Thus, drawing on the work of Foote (cited in Driver, 2007), a hypothetical can be constructed. When faced with the possibility of being in a position to save one drowning person (who is a stranger) on site A or five drowning people (who are also strangers) on site B, attending to the latter (site B) would be the clear (at least clear utilitarian) response. If the scenario is reframed such that the five drowning people can be saved only by driving over and killing someone in the road to reach them (which ultimately leads to the same outcome as not attending to site A), the decision is less likely to be clear-cut. The immediate and deliberate act of killing someone (even setting aside the legal implications) in pursuit of the "greater good" (in a utilitarian calculus) changes the situation. Moving back now to a care and technology angle, might care through remote monitoring and surveillance lead to a qualitatively different ethical approach by the carers? Thus, drawing on the previous hypothetical, the enquiry might be: are the care needs of a service user who is monitored remotely perceived in the same way as they would be if there were human contact, and will decisions over a course of action be different when the immediacy of care needs is filtered through a process of remote monitoring? (See Reynolds and Picard [2005] for a discussion about the use of affective computing in similar scenarios.)

Intuitionism in itself does not provide an adequately complete ethical framework but might usefully be employed in wider consideration about the use of technology. The inquiry here goes further; might this remote approach also facilitate easier decision making in the resource-limited context of social care for older people? Or if the care work force is reduced with the use of technological based substitutes, will numbers still be sufficient to address contingencies thrown up by the need to have remote care supplemented by actual physical intervention? Of course, if significant expenditure can be saved as a result of employing assistive technology and these savings are then redirected to enhance levels of care or service delivery that are targeted to those in most need, this might reasonably be put into (a very broad) calculus on beneficence (but might then be in tension with ethical codes around dignity and respect). Care services based on a human care workforce are also rationed, so this is not a clear-cut human versus technology dilemma. But the question remains: does the remoteness of the decision-making process where a centralized call center may be attending to multiple monitoring of service users make a difference to how action is prioritized or risk calculated, and by what calculation is a contingent workforce for intervention held in place in this arrangement?

CARE ASSESSING ACROSS PROFESSIONS

These ethical complexities and the difficulties of translating ethical decision making into a guide for frontline practitioners suggest that frameworks of ethical practice are in themselves, while important, of limited use and that virtue ethics (Banks & Gallagher, 2009). Perhaps both in combination with ethical codes and as a bridge across different professions that might be engaged in telecare assessing are relevant. This approach would link awareness of ethical codes and frameworks (which, in practice, are variously interpreted and variously employed) to the essential *virtuousness* of practitioners. Thus the difficulties of interpreting and employing ethical codes would be less problematic in the presence of the virtuous practitioner, who will be more likely to take the morally sound course of action by dint of his or her vocation and subsequent training. This might prove problematic unless there is a highly developed common understanding of what might constitute "virtue" in relation to care, especially in settings involving an increasing use of telecare technologies. This is made more complex by the advent of interprofessional working in the United Kingdom—and in particular Scotland—at the same time as telecare technologies are being introduced. This increasingly fluid world of assessing for care needs across professional boundaries (where education and training are different and different ethical codes are in play) may mean that recourse to virtue per se by dint of professional calling is open to question. There is now a literature that discusses the ethical issues in interprofessional working (see, for example, Leathard & McLaren, 2007) with more recent research looking at the frontline practice of interprofessional working where shared assessment tools are in use (Eccles, 2008). This latter research has noted inconsistencies across professions in the understanding of and consistency in obtaining consent with service users. But the thrust of recent policy has been to assume that common data sets are sufficiently straightforward to collect such that inconsistencies across professional disciplines will be minimal.

The interest here then is in the consistency of assessment across professions that assess care needs and recommend the use of telecare technologies. The approaches to care by different professional disciplines, ethical frameworks, and the use of these frameworks and the potential for vested interests in status quo care arrangements all suggest the potential for inconsistency of approaches to the use of telecare technologies. This is not, in itself, surprising; the impact of professional domains has long been recognized (Irvine, Kerridge, McPhee, & Freeman, 2002). How assessments are made and older people are care managed in the context of the use of technology across these domains would merit further research. The decision making processes may well be virtuous, but consistency of understanding of what constitutes virtue is open to question, as is just how virtuous decision making can be in the wider context of a culture of performance indicators that inform policy implementation.

There is a further complicating factor here, in that the Scottish Government's own preferred "partner" supplier of technology, Tunstall, offers packages of equipment, such that one element of equipment (a community alarm for example) would be automatically accompanied by further technology (for example, passive infrared monitoring) simultaneously installed in a recipient's home. This raises two considerations. First, it may not be cost-effective in the short term to oversupply equipment if it is not needed and the resources could be spent elsewhere. It might be cost-effective in the longer term, but this raises the second consideration. If the policy objective of the telecare strategy is to encourage autonomy and support independence, does not the provision of technology that is superfluous at a given point create the potential for *decreased* independence, and would care assessors across different professions necessarily see these dilemmas in the same light? The question of choice also accompanies the notion of independence and autonomy. If technological solutions prove to be the most cost-effective way of delivering care (for example, where packages of 24 hour care are required) in an era of increasingly rationed care budgets, are care recipients reasonably justified in opting for human care if that is indeed their chosen preference? And if technology offers the only care package that can reasonably be considered within fiscal constraints, will those recipients of care who are more resistant to using technology if it is installed, given their preference for human care services, be disadvantaged?

MANAGING THE RUBRIC

In discussing the ethics of management in health and social care, Girling (2007) notes the argument of Loughlin (2002) that the managerialist world of social services in the United Kingdom, with its emphasis on delivery and key performance indicators, lacks space beyond a rubric of ethical consideration for actual ethical practice. Girling summarizes this position thus: "Ethical reasoning requires the freedom of critical thought that is simply not available to managers" (Girling, 2007, p. 159), a position similarly discussed by Meagher and Parton (2004) around the use of "technical rational" rather "practical moral" decision making. Girling argues that the position is more complex than Loughlin suggests. He notes the difference between "cleverness" and "practical wisdom": managers may be good (that is, *clever*) at budgets and efficiency but "lack the practical wisdom to look for what the goals of the health and social care system should be in the first place" (p. 161). This manifests itself in the occasional absurdity of policy on the ground that it is designed to meet performance targets but patently does not serve the wider value bases in health and social care (for example, some prioritization of waiting lists in acute health care). Nonetheless, Girling (2007) argues that there is still scope for practical wisdom to be employed in practice settings. In this climate, managers face an ethical dilemma pitched between their own (perhaps virtue based) assessment of what might constitute a good outcome and the wider imperatives of meeting (and potentially being rewarded for meeting) performance indicators that might conflict with their virtuous judgement. The evaluation of telecare commissioned by the Scottish government introduces these caveats around the collation of figures about telecare activity (Scottish Government, 2009), and it is acknowledged that pursuing telecare technology in itself may offer incentives within the performance indicator framework (Beale, 2009).

There has also been a substantial injection of cash into the telecare program over the past two years, and this raises the question of what happens when this funding no longer exists. If care assessors deem that service users who have been in receipt of assistive technology would be better served in future by care services based not on technology but on human intervention, will there still be scope for this to happen? Fiscally, this may not be feasible as future care costing may be predicated on the anticipated use of technology; equally there may be a diminished supply of care workers, occasioned in part by the advent of the telecare program itself. Thus the reality of available resources and the policy paradigm currently being pursued may in themselves diminish the kind of discussion of ethical considerations raised in this paper simply by dint of options effectively being foreclosed. The need for practical wisdom here is clear, but the temptations of clever management strategies are, currently, positively reinforced.

CONCLUSION

The vision set out in the Scottish government's *Seizing the Opportunity: Telecare Strategy 2008–10*, noted at the start of this paper, sees Telecare as a future default option for care monitoring and an increased part of care delivery. This may well be laudable as a way of increasing independence and releasing funds; for example, for more intensive community-based care. But the discussion here suggests that there is a need for a more inquisitive ethical framework to accompany this process and for clearer safeguards to be employed across professional disciplines against cost reductions being a primary driver in the use of technology. As the pace of change in the use of assistive technology increases, the ability to display "practical wisdom" may become more difficult. Practical wisdom would need performance indicators that allowed for local discretion and an ethical framework that is more sophisticated. This framework need not necessarily extend to the assessment process but does need to be employed in evaluating and reflecting about the use of technology. Perhaps, above all, there needs to be more sensitivity to alternatives in the policy discourse; the challenges of demographic change may also serve as a basis for paradigm-shifting ways in which to reconfigure what care and caring relationships might look like in the 21st century. For all of the clear and well documented benefits of the use of telecare technology in human services, there needs now to be more debate about how it can best be ethically employed in a time of fiscal pressure and in settings where what is constituted as good care might have very different meanings for different user groups.

REFERENCES

Banks, S., & Gallagher, A. (2009). *Ethics in professional life: Virtues for health and social care*. Basingstoke: Palgrave Macmillan.

Barnes, M. (2006). *Caring and social justice*. Basingstoke: Palgrave MacMillan.

Beale, S. (2009). Evaluation of the Scottish government's telecare programme. Paper presented at the Connected Practice Symposium. Human Services in the Network Society: Changes, Challenges & Opportunities. The Institute for Advanced Studies, Glasgow 14–15, September 2009.

Beauchamp, L., & Childress, A. F. (2001). *Principles of biomedical ethics* (5th ed.). Oxford: Oxford University Press.

Blaschke, C., Freddolino, P., & Mullen, E. (2009). Ageing and technology: A review of the research literature. *British Journal of Social Work, 39*, 641–656.

Bowling, A., & Dieppe, P. (2005). What is successful aging and who should define it? *British Medical Journal, 331*, 1548–1551.

Care Services Improvement Partnership. (2005). *Telecare and ethics*. London: Crown Copyright.

Driver, J. (2007). *Ethics: The fundamentals*. Oxford: Blackwell.

Eccles, A. (2008). Singe shared assessment: The limits to "quick fix" implementation. *Journal of Integrated Care, 16*(1), 22–30.

Eccles, A. (2009). Some ethical considerations around the use of assistive technology. Paper presented at the Connected Practice Symposium. Human Services in the Network Society: Changes, Challenges & Opportunities. The Institute for Advanced Studies, Glasgow 14–15, September 2009.

European Union Public Health Information System. (2009). Population projections. Retrieved February 5, 2010, from http://www.euphix.org/object_document/o5116n27112.html

Freedland, J. (2009). The perfect gift? How about an end to loneliness—And not just at Christmas. Retrieved December 22, 2009, from http://www.guardian.co.uk/commentisfree/2009/dec/22/loneliness-at-christmas-public-services

Frisby, B. (2000). *ASTRID—A guide to using technology in dementia care*. London: Hawker.

General Register Office for Scotland. (2009). Projected population of Scotland. Retrieved February 6, 2010, from http://www.gro-scotland.gov.uk/statistics/publications-and-data/popproj/projected-population-of-scotland-2008-based/list-of-tables.html

Girling, J. (2007). Ethics and the management of health and social care. In A. Leathard & S. McLaren (Eds.), *Ethics: Contemporary challenges in health and social care* (pp. 157–168). Bristol: Policy Press.

Hanson, J., Osipovic, D., & Percival, J. (2009). Making sense of sensors. In B. Loader, M. Hardey & L. Keeble (Eds.), *Digital welfare for the third age* (pp. 91–111). London: Routledge.

Held, V. (2006). *The ethics of care: Personal, political, global*. New York: Oxford University Press.

Irvine, R., Kerridge, I., McPhee, J., & Freeman, S. (2002). Interprofessionalism and ethics: Consensus or clash of cultures? *Journal of Interprofessional Care, 16*(3), 199–210.

Johnstone, J. (2007). Technology as empowerment: A capability approach to computer ethics. *Ethics and Information Technology, 9*, 73–87.

Leathard, A., & McLaren, S. (Eds.) (2007). *Ethics: Contemporary challenges in health and social care.* Bristol: Policy Press.

Loader, B., Hardey, M., & Keeble, L. (Eds.) (2009). *Digital welfare for the third age.* London: Routledge.

Loughlin, M. (2002). *Ethics, management and mythology.* Abingdon: Radcliffe Medical Press.

Lowe, C. (2009). Beyond telecare: The future of independent living. *Journal of Assistive Technologies, 3*(1), 21–23.

Lymbery, M. (2005). *Social work with older people.* London: Sage.

McCreadie, C., & Tinker, A. (2005). The acceptability of assistive technology to older people. *Ageing and Society, 25*, 91–110.

Meagher, G., & Parton, N. (2004). Modernising social work and the ethics of care. *Social Work and Society, 2*(1), 10–27.

Means, R., Richards, S., & Smith, R. (2008). *Community care* (4th ed). Basingstoke: Palgrave.

Morbey, H., Smith, R., & Means, R. (2002). *From community care to market care: The development of welfare serves for older people.* Oxford: Polity.

Mort, M., Roberts, C., & Milligan, C. (2009). Ageing, technology and the home: A critical project. *European Journal of Disability Research, 3*, 85–89.

Noddings, N. (1984). *Caring: A feminine approach to ethics and moral education.* Berkeley: University of California Press.

Page, R. (2007). *Revisiting the welfare state.* Buckingham: Open University Press.

Phillips, J. (2007). *Care.* Oxford: Polity.

Pols, J., & Moser, I. (2009). Cold technologies versus warm care? On affective and social relations with and through care technologies. *European Journal of Disability Research, 3*, 159–178.

Ratto, M. (2007). Ethics of seamless infrastructures: Resources and future directions. *International Review of Information Ethics, 8*, 21–27.

Reynolds, C., & Pickard, R. (2005). Evaluation of affective computing systems from a dimensional metaethical position. Proceedings of the 1st Augmented Cognition Conference, in conjunction with the 11th International Conference on Human–Computer Interaction. Retrieved February 2, 2010, from http://citeseerx.ist.psu.edu/viewdoc/download?doi=10.1.1.68.733&rep=rep1&type=pdf

Scottish Government. (2007). Telecare factsheet: Ethics and assessment. Retrieved 10 March 2009 from http://www.jitscotland.org.uk/downloads/1208876248-78-Ethics%20&%20Assessment.pdf.

Scottish Government. (2008a). *Seizing the opportunity: Telecare strategy 2008–10.* Edinburgh: Crown Copyright.

Scottish Government. (2008b). *Telecare in Scotland: Benchmarking the present, embracing the future.* Edinburgh: Crown Copyright.

Scottish Government. (2009). *Evaluation of the Telecare Development Programme: Final report.* Edinburgh: Crown Copyright.

Sommerville, J. (2003). Juggling law, ethics and intuition: Practical answers to awkward questions. *Journal of Medical Ethics, 29*, 281–286.

Steyaert, J., & Gould, N. (2009). Social work and the changing face of the digital divide. *British Journal of Social Work, 39*(4), 740–753.

Tao, J., & Drover, G. (1997). Chinese and Western notions of need. *Critical Social Policy, 17*, 5–25.

Taylor, J. R., Groleau, C., Heaton, L., & Van Every, E. (2000). *The computerization of work: A communication perspective.* Thousand Oaks, CA: Sage.

Tinker, A. (1997). *Older people in modern society.* London: Longman.

Townsend, P. (2006). Policies for the aged in the 21st century: More "structured dependency" or the realisation of human rights? *Ageing and Society, 26*(2), 161–179.

Tronto, J. (1993). *Moral boundaries: A political argument for an ethic of care.* London: Routeledge.

Tunstall. (2009). *Support for carers: Solutions for independent living.* Retrieved February 2, 2010, from http://www.tunstall.co.uk/assets/literature/Carers%20guide.pdf

Wilmot, S. (1997). *The ethics of community care.* London: Cassell.

The Initial Evaluation of the Scottish Telecare Development Program

SOPHIE BEALE, PAUL TRUMAN,
DIANA SANDERSON, and JEN KRUGER

York Health Economics Consortium, University of York, York, UK

In 2006 the Scottish Government provided just over £8 million to help 32 health and social care partnerships to develop telecare services. This paper presents a summary of the 2007–2008 evaluation of the Scottish Telecare Development. This evaluation focused on measuring overall program progress toward eight predefined Scottish Telecare Development objectives. Results indicate that the initial investment has resulted in significant savings to the health and social care sectors. Additionally, telecare provides opportunities to promote independence and improve the quality of life of service users and their informal carers. However, some caution needs to be taken in interpreting the findings as results are based on self-reported performance from partnerships, and many of the reported monetary "savings" are actually efficiency savings and are unlikely, in practice, to be cash-releasing.

INTRODUCTION

Information and communication technology are playing an increasingly large role in our everyday lives. Historic ways of communicating (such as face-to-face meetings and the exchange of letters) have been joined by methods that include phone calls, video conferences, texts, and e-mails. Recently, options have been further increased by the emergence of methods including discussion boards, blogs, and social networking. Similarly, with the development of computer memory and processing power, the way information is collected, stored, and used has change from necessarily being quite simple to a stage where boundaries seem to be limited by human imagination. Through using these and other new technologies, industries are adapting the services and products they offer and are changing the way they interact with their customers. Advances in information and communication technology are increasingly being employed in the delivery of health and social care. Where these are used in the remote interface between patients/clients and clinicians/care staff they are often known as telemedicine, telehealth, or telecare.

The Scottish Telecare Development Programme (TDP) was launched in August 2006 with the following aim: "To help more people in Scotland live at home for longer, with safety and security, by promoting the use of telecare in Scotland through the provision of a development fund and associated support" (Joint Improvement Team, 2006a). The TDP adopted a definition of telecare taken from the "Shared Vocabulary" agreed and published by the Scottish Government:

> Telecare is the remote or enhanced delivery of health and social services to people in their own homes by means of telecommunications and computerized systems. Telecare usually refers to equipment and detectors that provide continuous, automatic and remote monitoring of care needs, emergencies and lifestyle changes, using information and communication technology (ICT) to trigger human responses, or shut down equipment to prevent hazards. (Joint Improvement Team, 2006b; Scottish Government, 2008)

The TDP, which is managed by the Scottish Executive's Joint Improvement Team (JIT), has eight objectives. These are to:

1. Reduce the number of avoidable emergency admissions and readmissions to hospital
2. Increase the speed of discharge from hospital once clinical need is met
3. Reduce the use of care homes
4. Improve the quality of life of users of telecare services
5. Reduce the pressure on informal carers
6. Extend the range of people assisted by telecare services in Scotland

7. Achieve efficiencies (cash releasing or time releasing) from investment in telecare

8. Support effective procurement to ensure that telecare services grow as quickly as possible. (Joint Improvement Team, 2006b)

JIT received just over £8 million in the summer of 2006 to help 32 Scottish health and social care partnerships to develop telecare services during 2006–2008. Nominal allocations to each partnership were based on their populations, and funds were distributed by JIT on receipt of satisfactory applications outlining partnership intentions. A total of £6,832,312 was allocated to partnerships in this period.

Researchers at York Health Economics Consortium (YHEC), a health economics research and consultancy company owned by the University of York, were commissioned by JIT to carry out an evaluation of the TDP. The evaluation focused primarily on considering the extent to which the eight TDP objectives were achieved during 2006–2008. This paper summarizes how the TDP performed against the objectives and discusses some of the issues faced by the evaluation. The full evaluation report can be found on the JIT Web site (Beale, Sanderson, & Kruger, 2009).

METHODS

The evaluation considered the impact of the TDP as a whole rather than the performance of individual projects. It comprised three main elements: use of data provided by the partnerships via quarterly returns, postal questionnaires that were distributed to service users and informal carers, and case studies.

Quarterly Returns

Partnerships in receipt of TDP funding were required to submit information on performance toward TDP objectives and locally identified outcomes and efficiencies to JIT on a quarterly basis. The quarterly returns asked them to evaluate individual user-level data to determine whether the presence of telecare had resulted in improvements in care. In terms of national objectives, partnerships were asked to consider whether telecare had resulted in any of the following:

- Reduction in emergency admissions to hospital
- Reduction in delayed discharges from hospital
- Reduction in care home admissions

Additionally, they were asked, based on local knowledge (including clinical knowledge) of the circumstances of individuals who were in receipt of telecare, to provide an estimate of the duration of each admission or delayed discharge avoided. Where only the numbers of admissions or discharges avoided were supplied, the researchers derived an estimate of the length of such episodes from aggregated national data. Estimates of the financial savings resulting from avoided admissions and discharges were derived by applying unit costs to health and care home admissions. Where local costs were not available costs were extracted from the "Costs Book 2008" (ISD Scotland, 2009) or estimated based on data submitted by other partnerships.

Partnerships were also asked to provide details about local outcomes and efficiencies (e.g., sleepover care, home check visits, waking night cover). The other main areas covered in the quarterly returns were the demographic details of new telecare clients and information about the telecare equipment procurement process.

User and Carer Questionnaires

Two questionnaires were developed (one for users and the other for their informal carers). The user questionnaire was designed to collect information on users' perceptions of the impact of telecare on their health and quality of life. The carer questionnaire explored the change in pressure on informal carers. The questionnaires were distributed toward the end of the evaluation period. In some instances partnerships distributed the questionnaires along with additional questions that sought information to inform local telecare related planning decisions.

Case Studies

Five partnerships, implementing a range of different projects, were invited to participate as case studies. The case studies provided a detailed assessment of how TDP funding had been used to help people to live at home for longer with safety and security. They also provided detailed feedback on local experiences of developing and implementing telecare services. Site visits allowed the researchers to carry out face-to-face interviews with a range of local managers and operational staff, meet some service users and their carers, and see local facilities for demonstrating relevant equipment.

RESULTS

Quarterly returns covering the 2007–2008 financial year were received from a total of 32 partnerships. Not all partnerships were operational for the full year due to delays in implementing services and, in total, only 25 partnerships were able to provide four returns during 2007–2008. The quantitative findings presented in the following sections are based on information from all the submitted returns.

Telecare Recipient Population Characteristics

A total of approximately £6.8 million was allocated to partnerships during 2006–2007 and 2007–2008 to support the implementation of their telecare projects. Initially, partnerships planned to implement a total of 73 projects. Of these, six were operational by the end of the 2006–2007 financial year (i.e., April 2007, the start of the evaluation period), and 51 were operational by the end of the 2007–2008 financial year (i.e., April 2008, the end of the evaluation period). Most of the projects were designed with older people in mind and focused on extending and developing existing telecare services.

During the 2007–2008 financial year 7,902 people were supplied with TDP-funded equipment, although not all had the equipment for the full year. At the end of 2007–2008 there were 7,487 clients in receipt of TDP-funded equipment. The numbers ceasing to use telecare were relatively small and, in many cases, are easily explained (e.g., telecare service was provided to address a short-term, acute need, or user died).

Overall, 62.4% of new clients were female, 84.5% were White, and 85.0% were aged 65 years or over. The two most frequently cited reasons for providing telecare to a client were to "minimize client risk" (69.0%) and to "promote client independence" (11.1%). There is a certain amount of overlap between these two categories as minimizing client risk will help to promote client independence. The main reasons for receipt of telecare are displayed in Table 1.

Impact of Telecare on Emergency Admissions and Readmissions

Table 2 shows the number of emergency admissions that partnerships reported were avoided during 2007–2008. The number increased over the course of the study, mainly as a result of the increase in the number of partnerships that implemented telecare solutions. Partnerships estimated that a total of over 1,200 hospital admissions were avoided as a result of telecare projects supported by the TDP. Partnership estimates of the duration of avoided admissions ranged from 2 days to 30 days. These admissions were estimated to be associated with over 13,000 bed days (the equivalent to 38 beds, assuming full occupancy).

Nearly three quarters (74.2%) of the bed days saved were associated with care provided to older people, 8.4% to clients with mental health issues and 5.7% to those with dementia (figures were not available, but many of those with dementia are likely to be elderly).

Impact of Telecare on Facilitating Hospital Discharge

In addition to emergency admissions avoided, partnerships also reported that telecare had facilitated faster discharge for many users who were hospitalized. The evaluation findings suggest that over 500 delayed discharges

TABLE 1 Main Reasons for Receiving Telecare

Reason	Number (%) of individuals
Minimize client risk	5,453 (69.0)
Promote client independence	881 (11.1)
Prevent long-term admission to care home	289 (3.7)
Facilitate hospital discharge	309 (3.9)
Reduce risk of hospital admission/readmission	462 (5.8)
Monitor client to assess longer-term needs	209 (2.6)
Part of intermediate care package	142 (1.8)
Carer support	137 (1.7)
Unknown	20 (0.3)
Total	7,902

TABLE 2 Cumulative Progress Toward Reducing Hospital Bed Days Through Reducing the Number of Avoidable Emergency Admissions and Readmissions

	2007–2008			
	Quarter 1	Quarter 2	Quarter 3	Quarter 4
Number of partnerships (projects)	7 (7)	9 (9)	16 (18)	18 (22)
Hospital admissions avoided (cumulative)	210	321	761	1,220
Hospital bed days avoided (cumulative)	508	1,165	8,203	13,870

were avoided as a result of telecare, leading to an estimated saving of over 5,000 bed days, as shown in Table 3. These discharges were facilitated by the availability of increased monitoring of patients in home care settings.

Nearly three quarters (73.8%) of the bed days saved were associated with care provided to older people, 13.2% to clients whose category was not provided, 7.1% to those with a physical disability, and 5.0% to clients with dementia (figures were not available, but many of those with a physical disability and dementia are likely to be elderly).

Impact of Telecare on the Use of Care Homes

Responses received from 23 of the partnerships suggested that telecare resulted in avoided admissions to care homes. In some cases telecare

TABLE 3 Cumulative Progress toward Reducing Hospital Bed Days Through Facilitating Hospital Discharges

	2007–2008			
	Quarter 1	Quarter 2	Quarter 3	Quarter 4
Number of partnerships (projects)	8 (8)	13 (13)	16 (17)	20 (21)
Hospital discharges facilitated (cumulative)	48	111	408	517
Hospital bed days saved (cumulative)	1,033	2,197	3,991	5,668

TABLE 4 Cumulative Progress Toward Reducing the Number of Care Home Bed Days

	2007–2008			
	Quarter 1	Quarter 2	Quarter 3	Quarter 4
Number of partnerships (projects)	10 (12)	14 (16)	19 (22)	23 (26)
Care home admissions avoided (cumulative)	63	153	332	518
Care home bed days avoided (cumulative)	5,129	13,727	28,392	61,993

facilitated the avoidance of admission to long-term care, and in other cases it led to the avoidance of short-term respite admissions. In total, partnerships estimated that 518 admissions to care homes had been avoided over the course of the evaluation. Modeling (based on information supplied by the partnerships) indicated that these were associated with the avoidance of a significant length of stay, equating to in excess of 60,000 bed days over the course of the evaluation (equivalent to c.170 care home beds, assuming full occupancy). A summary of the impact of telecare on admissions to care homes is displayed in Table 4.

Nearly half (48.9%) of the care home bed days saved were associated with telecare clients whose underlying condition was unknown, 29.1% were associated with clients with dementia, and 16.9% to older clients.

Estimated Monetary Savings

Applying appropriate unit costs to the bed days saved allows an estimate of the financial impact of the TDP to be generated. Table 5 shows the estimated financial savings for each quarter, including those that resulted from local

TABLE 5 Estimated Financial Savings Resulting from Telecare Projects

	2007–2008				
	Quarter 1	Quarter 2	Quarter 3	Quarter 4	Total
Total savings					
Quarterly financial savings	£1,125,071	£1,875,188	£4,317,738	£3,833,194	£11,151,191
Contributing Savings					
TDP objectives					
Increased speed of discharge	£434,975	£307,354	£558,861	£430,755	£1,731,945
Unplanned hospital admissions	£156,809	£311,389	£1,549,735	£1,325,534	£3,343,467
Care home admissions	£202,827	£505,454	£1,287,828	£1,425,512	£3,421,621
Local savings					
Nights of sleepover care	£25,450	£118,450	£211,999	£201,220	£557,119
Home check visits	£304,810	£632,541	£421,955	£436,733	£1,796,039
Waking night care	£200	–	£287,360	£13,440	£301,000

partnership efficiencies. The cumulative savings associated with the TDP are estimated to be in excess of £11 million. The majority of savings result from avoiding unplanned hospital and care home admissions, although notable savings also resulted from a reduced demand for home check visits and the reduction in delayed discharges.

Impact of Telecare on the Quality of Life of Service Users

Service user questionnaires were returned by 461 users in 19 partnerships. Just over half of the respondents felt that their current quality of life was either "good" or "very good." About three fifths (60.5%) of the respondents felt that their current quality of life was either "a bit better" or "much better" than before their telecare equipment was installed, about a third (34.6%) thought that it had "stayed the same," and less than 1 in 20 (4.9%) felt that it was worse.

In terms of telecare's impact on specific aspects likely to affect users' quality of life,

- over half (55.2%) felt that their health had not changed, while slightly more than half of the other respondents (27.1% of the total) thought that their health had improved;
- almost all (93.3%) respondents felt safer;
- over two thirds (69.7%) felt more independent;
- very few (3.5%) felt lonelier;
- four fifths (82.3%) either "disagreed" or "strongly disagreed" that they felt more anxious and stressed;
- most (87.2%) thought that their families now worried less about them;
- about two fifths (40.8%) felt that their equipment had not affected the amount of help they needed from their family, while about one third (32.8%) felt that they needed less help.

Respondents were generally very positive about telecare services, and overall, telecare services have had significant positive impacts on the quality of life of service users.

Impact of Telecare on Informal Carers

Carer questionnaires were returned by 301 carers in 17 partnerships. Almost half (48.3%) of these were completed by daughters (34.1%) or sons (14.3%). A slightly higher proportion of respondents currently found their caring role either "quite stressful" or "very stressful" (46.5%) than found it "not really stressful" or "not at all stressful" (36.9%). About three quarters (74.3%) of respondents felt that the telecare equipment had reduced the pressures on them by reducing their stress levels, and fewer than 1 in 20 (4.3%) felt that their stress levels had increased. The main reasons for changes in respondents' stress levels seem in part to depend on

- the characteristics of the cared for person;
- the type(s) of equipment installed;
- the type of responder service.

The time spent with the cared for person had remained "about the same" for approximately three quarters (73.0%) of the respondents (with similar proportions spending "more time" and "less time" with the cared for persons). Respondents generally felt that the equipment gave them peace of mind as they worried less (e.g., about falls). Overall, many respondents were very positive about the telecare service and also very grateful for it.

Effective Procurement

To promote the effective procurement of telecare equipment by partnerships, JIT recommended that they should use the established National Framework Agreement (NFA) with the NHS (National Health Service) Purchasing and Supply Agency (PASA). Thirteen partnerships used PASA for all purchases, 4 used if for some purchases, and 11 did not use it at all (although some used it indirectly). The main reason partnerships gave for not using the NFA was that they were able to purchase equipment more cheaply through alternative mechanisms. Those partnerships that had used PASA had experienced relatively few problems with the system.

Lessons Learned from the Case Studies

The five selected case study sites reported a variety of experiences during 2006–2008. Attempts were made to include geographically diverse populations, covering both urban and rural environments, to explore the impact that geography can have on access to care and the potential role of telecare in this respect. It is, however, acknowledged that the findings from a sample of five case studies are not necessarily generalizable.

A number of lessons for others interested in developing or extending telecare services can be learned from the experiences of these case study sites, including the following:

- Sufficient dedicated managerial input is necessary.
- A local "champion," preferably working at senior officer level, is important.
- Do not be too ambitious when setting up projects using telecare and set realistic timescales for their development.

- A significant amount of time is usually required to develop a positive local culture toward telecare and to "win people's hearts and minds."
- Recognize the time required to provide appropriate training to a wide range of staff from many health, social care, and housing-related settings (which can be greatly assisted by a demonstration house or similar).
- It is likely to take up to a year of preparatory work before telecare clients can be recruited.
- Even if basic packages of telecare are used, it will be necessary to have some flexibility to ensure that people's specific needs are met.
- Telecare equipment can have a dramatic effect on the lives of some people, especially older people (including those with dementia) and people with long-term conditions and learning disabilities.
- Informal carers can also benefit greatly from telecare equipment.
- A 24/7 professional responder service is very beneficial and popular (providing it is practical to deliver such a service—it may sometimes be necessary to consider some imaginative forms for delivering such a service).
- The partnerships see telecare as part of a package of services helping people remain in their own homes, and the specific financial effects due, for example, to any resultant increased demand for other services, are not being monitored.

DISCUSSION

The economic findings of the evaluation of the Scottish TDP are encouraging. The summary results suggest that the initial funding to partnerships of approximately £6.8 million in the TDP has resulted in savings to the Scottish health and social care budgets of approximately £11 million during 2007–2008. From an economic perspective, the findings suggest that the allocation of funding to the TDP was an effective use of resources, generating a significant return on investment. In addition to this, there are undoubtedly some further efficiency savings in terms of the planning and delivery of care that have not been quantified in this analysis. Although these findings are based on data collected over a single year following the commencement of most of the TDP funded telecare projects, they suggest that the widespread adoption of telecare may have the potential to lead to modest reductions in bed numbers both in health and social care settings.

Previous studies have produced positive findings on the financial impact of telecare services. The evaluation of the West Lothian initiative to provide free telecare to support individuals with dementia was estimated to have avoided admissions to long-term care resulting in telecare saving approximately £150 per user per week (Bowes & McColgan, 2006). However, the majority of previous studies that have sought to capture the economic impact of telecare have either considered the impact of a specific technology used in a single indication (Clark, Inglis, McAlister, Cleland, & Stewart, 2007) or uptake of a range of telecare interventions in a relatively small population (Aleszewski & Cappello, 2006). Attempts are currently underway, through the Whole-System Demonstrator Programme, to explore the impact of large-scale uptake of telecare and telehealth in England (Department of Health, 2009). Large scale controlled trials are being undertaken at three sites to determine whether widespread adoption can lead to improved outcomes and financial savings, with a view to providing definitive evidence on the value of mainstream adoption of telecare and telehealth.

However, some caution needs to be taken in interpreting these findings. The results are based on self-reported performance from partnerships in receipt of TDP funding. While partnerships were provided with training on how to complete the quarterly reports, some partnerships continued to have significant difficulties in providing meaningful estimates of the impact of the TDP on health and social care resources. As such, there is expected to be some uncertainty in the estimates of bed days saved. In addition to this, the approach adopted is subject to some degree of responder bias; that is, partnerships may have an incentive to over- or underestimate the impact of the TDP funding to secure future funding. Finally, it should be noted that many of the reported monetary "savings" are actually efficiency savings and are unlikely to be cash-releasing in practice. For example, reductions in care home admissions may be meaningless if such services are purchased on a block-contract basis. Any return on investment calculations are urged to take this latter point into consideration. Findings from the TDP evaluation, which are based on a relatively small number of telecare users spread across a wide geographical area, suggest that securing funding for telecare on the basis that it will be cost saving to the health service is unlikely to be a successful approach in the short- to medium-term as health care payers fail to see net financial savings materialize.

Limitations of the Study Design

The evaluation adopted a pragmatic research design that attempted to work with data that were already available in partnerships or which partnerships should easily be able to generate. This resulted in a methodology which relied heavily on the expertise and experience within partnerships to accurately report the impact of telecare interventions. For reasons of equity it was deemed undesirable to randomly assign individuals to telecare interventions. Similarly, due to the range of interventions considered in the program and its national reach, it was not possible to identify meaningful control groups from regions outside the program. As a result, it was neither possible nor desirable to undertake any form of randomized or nonrandomized comparative analysis of the impact of the TDP.

An alternative approach considered was to capture historic user-level resource use data that could be compared with data captured prospectively following the introduction of telecare. While this "before and after" approach would have provided some estimate of the incremental impact of telecare on individual users, this study design was also deemed to be unsuitable on two grounds. First, user-level health and social care data could not be accessed in real-time during the course of the study and, as such, this approach would have significantly extended the evaluation period and delayed reporting. Second, this approach was also recognized as having limitations as historic resource use may be a poor indicator of future events for many of the users of telecare. Many of the interventions supported by the program are intended to support users and carers following an acute event that leads to an increased reliance on formal care, such as a stroke or the onset of dementia. In these instances, an individual user's history of use of residential care, respite care, and hospital admissions may be relatively low prior to the event but increase sharply following the event. Similarly, many users may have progressive illnesses, meaning that the use of formal care will be expected to increase over time.

Implications for the Further Adoption of Telecare

By acknowledging the limitations inherent in the evaluation of the TDP and discussing alternative approaches that were considered, it is hoped that evaluations of future attempts to support widespread adoption of telecare might build on the methods adopted herein. While randomized controlled trials of individual telecare technologies are undoubtedly useful in providing evidence of efficacy, their external validity to a broader population characterized by complex needs is limited. Furthermore, using randomized controlled trials to evaluate the impact of widespread adoption of a range of telecare technologies in practice is neither feasible nor desirable, as such trials are unlikely to be able to accommodate the heterogeneity of users, interventions, and settings that is inherent in the application of telecare in practice.

In endorsing the use of more pragmatic study approaches, it is important that such approaches include some form of control arm or comparative data. Some form of managed adoption of telecare throughout a region would allow for benchmarking of practice against similar populations or similar organizations to determine whether new technologies are fulfilling their promise to improve efficiency. "Risk-sharing" approaches, as increasingly applied to pharmaceuticals (Cook, Vernon, & Manning, 2008), may be an appropriate means of addressing the desire for increased adoption coupled with the need for more evidence on performance. By incorporating an evaluation alongside uptake and monitoring against prespecified performance measures, it should be possible to determine whether further, more widespread adoption is warranted.

Finally, those responsible for commissioning telecare services should not lose sight of the primary intention of such services. It is easy to focus on the potential efficiency savings of telecare, particularly when health and social care resources are increasingly scarce. While many telecare interventions undoubtedly have the potential to lead to reduced use of secondary care and social care resources, it should be emphasized that the primary objective of telecare is to support users and ultimately lead to improvements in health and well-being. Our findings suggest that telecare interventions are valued by users and carers and reflect previous research that has suggested that such interventions can lead to improvements in patients' perceptions of the quality of care they receive and ultimately their quality of life (Brownsell, Blackburn, & Hawley, 2008). These outcomes are not always consistent with efficiency gains or monetary savings, and health care planners are encouraged to adopt a realistic view about the potential financial implications of the adoption of telecare rather than a "spend-to-save" approach.

Conclusion

The evaluation of the Scottish Telecare Development Programme suggests that the initial investment has resulted in significant savings to the health and social care sectors and has improved the levels of patient and carer satisfaction with their care. These findings suggest that there may be value in the more widespread adoption of telecare. However, health care planners are encouraged to adopt a realistic view toward savings as many of the reported monetary "savings" are actually efficiency savings and are unlikely, in practice, to be cash-releasing.

REFERENCES

Aleszewski, A., & Cappello, R. (2006). Piloting telecare in Kent County Council: The key lessons. Final report 2006. *Kent: Centre for Health Services Studies, University of Kent.* Retrieved February 12, 2010, from http://www.kent.ac.uk/chss/docs/telecare_final_report.pdf

Beale, S., Sanderson, D., & Kruger, J. (2009). Evaluation of the telecare development programme: Final report. *Joint Improvement Team, Scottish Government.* Retrieved February 12, 2010, from http://www.jitscotland.org.uk/action-areas/telecare-in-scotland/telecare-publications/

Bowes, A., & McColgan, G. (2006). Smart technology and community care for older people: Innovation in West Lothian, Scotland. *Age Concern Scotland.* Retrieved February 12, 2010, from www.ageconcernandhelptheagedscotland.org.uk/documents/114

Brownsell, S., Blackburn, S., & Hawley, M. S. (2008). An evaluation of second and third generation telecare services in older people's housing. *Journal of Telecare and Telemedicine, 14*(1), 8–12.

Clark, R. A., Inglis, S. C., McAlister, F. A., Cleland, J. G. F., & Stewart, S. (2007). Telemonitoring or structured telephone support programmes for patients with chronic heart failure: A systematic review and meta-analysis. *British Medical Journal, 334*(7600), 942–945.

Cook, J. P., Vernon, J. A., & Manning, R. (2008). Pharmaceutical risk-sharing agreements. *Pharmacoeconomics, 26*(7), 551–556.

Department of Health. (2009). The whole systems demonstrators: An overview of telecare and telehealth. Retrieved February 12, 2010, from http://www.dh.gov.uk/dr_consum_dh/groups/dh_digitalassets/documents/digitalasset/dh_100947.pdf

ISD Scotland. (2009). Costs book 2008. Retrieved February 12, 2010, from http://www.isdscotland.org/isd/6058.html

Joint Improvement Team. (2006a). National telecare development programme: Glossary of terms and conditions. Retrieved February 12, 2010, from http://www.jitscotland.org.uk/action-areas/telecare-in-scotland

Joint Improvement Team. (2006b). Proposal: Telecare development programme. Retrieved February 12, 2010, from http://www.jitscotland.org.uk/downloads/1208770769-Telecare%20Development%20Programme%20Proposal%20May%202006.pdf

Scottish Government. (2008). Shared vocabulary. Retrieved February 12, 2010, from http://www.scotland.gov.uk/Topics/Health/care/EandA/vocab

Privacy, Social Network Sites, and Social Relations

DAVID J. HOUGHTON and ADAM N. JOINSON

University of Bath, Bath, UK

With the growth of the Internet comes a growth in a ubiquitous networked society. Common Web 2.0 applications include a rapidly growing trend for social network sites. Social network sites typically converged different relationship types into one group of "friends." However, with such vast interconnectivity, convergence of relationships, and information sharing by individual users comes an increased risk of privacy violations. We asked a small sample of participants to discuss what friendship and privacy meant to them and to give examples of a privacy violation they had experienced. A thematic analysis was conducted on the interviews to determine the issues discussed by the participants. Many participants experienced privacy issues using the social network site Facebook. The results are presented here and discussed in relation to online privacy concerns, notably social network site privacy concerns and managing such information.

INTRODUCTION

The increased prevalence and use of information communication technologies (ICTs) have transformed many people's lives in terms of how they work, form, and maintain social relations and plan and use leisure time (Anawati & Craig, 2006). This rise in a networked society has not been without concern about, variously, the mental well-being of Internet users (Kraut et al., 2002; Kraut et al., 1998), the "pseudo" nature of communities and friendships forged online (Jones, 1995), dangers to children of either the content or time spent online (Hasebrink, Livingstone, Haddon, & Ólafsson, 2009), and loss of social capital and trust in a virtual workplace (Handy, 1995). The work in the present paper addresses another concern raised frequently in discussions of the networked society: privacy. More specifically, we are interested in how privacy can be negotiated by people in social network sites (SNS) such as Facebook.

Social network sites typically share three common elements. They allow individuals to "construct a public or semi-public profile within a bounded system, articulate a list of other users with whom they share a connection, and view and traverse their list of connections and those made by others within the system" (Boyd & Ellison, 2007, p. 211). A number of studies have demonstrated that the large-scale mobilization in Facebook is sparked by the opportunity to connect and communicate with people one has met or befriended off line (Ellison, Steinfeld, & Lampe, 2007; Golder, Wilkinson, & Huberman, 2007; Joinson, 2008; Lampe, Ellison, & Steinfield, 2006) and to a lesser degree by the ability to investigate new others (Ellison et al., 2007; Joinson, 2008; Lampe et al., 2006). A range of content-sharing uses sustains these motivations, such as posting photographs, using applications, and changing the status update (Joinson, 2008). At a macro level, the intensity of using Facebook to maintain off line ties is related to different kinds of social capital formed within the off line community (Ellison et al., 2007).

Facebook, in addition to personal use and for keeping up with old friends (Joinson, 2008), is often used between colleagues, and managing such conflicting spheres can prove difficult (Binder, Howes, & Sutcliffe, 2009; DiMicco & Millen, 2007). Examples of violations are often seen in the media. For example, an employee in England was reported to have been dismissed because she wrote that her job was "totally boring" on her Facebook status ("Facebook Remark Teenager Is Fired," 2009).

Social Networking and Privacy

In 2008, Internet access in the UK had increased to include 65% (16.46 million) of all households, an increase of 1.23 million since 2007. Great Britain has seen an increase of an average 1 million households per year since 2004 (UK Office of National Statistics, 2008).

Currently, Facebook has more than 350 million active users. Fifty percent of these users log in daily. There are more that 2.5 billion photos uploaded each month, with more than 3.5 billion pieces of content shared each week (including Web links, news stories, blog posts, notes, photo albums etc.) (Facebook, 2010). There are currently more than 70 translations of the site available, with 70% of Facebook users coming from outside of the United States (Facebook, 2010). The average user has 130 friends, sends 8 friend requests per month, is a member of 12 groups, and spends more than

55 minutes per day on the site (Facebook, 2010). As of December 2009, Facebook accounts for 7% of all time spent online in the United States (Lipsman, 2010). This increased use of social network sites has led to increased concerns about users' privacy not only in terms of the data collected and used by the organization but also in light of the possible impact of mass sharing of personal information on social relations.

PRIVACY AND NEW TECHNOLOGY

Westin (1967) defines privacy as "the claim of individuals, groups, or institutions to determine for themselves when, how and to what extent information about them is communicated to others" (p. 7). According to Westin, it is achieved through four main methods: "the voluntary and temporary withdrawal of a person from general society through physical or psychological means, either in a state of solitude or small group intimacy or, when among large groups, in a condition of anonymity or reserve" (Westin, 1967, p. 7).

Altman (1975, p. 24) defines privacy as "the selective control of access to the self" and argues that privacy is achieved through the regulation of social interaction. Both Westin's and Altman's theories have stimulated much of the research and theory development of privacy (Margulis, 2003). However, despite many attempts to create a synthesis of the existing literature in this area (e.g., Parent, 1983; Schoeman, 1984), a unified and simple account of privacy has yet to emerge. Because of this, more recent approaches have tended to focus on the different dimensions of privacy. For instance, Burgoon, Parrott, le Poire, & Kelley (1989) distinguish four dimensions of privacy and define it using these dimensions as "the ability to control and limit *physical, interactional, psychological* and *informational* access to the self or one's group" (p. 132). DeCew (1997) also reflects the multidimensional nature of privacy in her definition, which distinguishes three dimensions: *informational, accessibility,* and *expressive privacy.* According to Schatz Byford (1996), "At no time have privacy issues taken on greater significance than in recent years, as technological developments have led to the emergence of an 'information society' capable of gathering, storing and disseminating increasing amounts of data about individuals" (p. 1).

While the underlying concept of privacy is not new, modern technological advancements have meant that privacy concerns have evolved. New ICTs have transformed our ability to collect, aggregate, and share data. Modern technology has the ability and power, particularly in comparison to the precomputer era, to capture, store, aggregate, redistribute, and use data from individual users (Sparck Jones, 2003). Sparck Jones (2003) discusses the permanence and vast quantity of the records held in such databases. Noting that the owner of this information is often unaware of, or at least unconnected to, its storage and utilization, she argues that such ubiquitous data collection is harmful to personal privacy and autonomy, regardless of whether individuals differ on what they determine is private (Sparck Jones, 2003). The resultant harms of privacy violations may be both physical (e.g., bodily privacy) and psychological (e.g., fear of surveillance) (Altman, 1975; Joinson, 2009; Krueger, 2005; Solove, 2006; Warren & Brandeis, 1890; Westin, 1967). Solove (2007) reflects on this with the modern story of "dog poop girl." "Dog poop girl," as she is now known, was subject to the use of her image by a fellow train passenger after she had refused to clean up her dog's excrement on an underground train. The unauthorized use of her image by a fellow passenger resulted in widespread dissemination. Had it not been for the ease of dissemination and search ability offered by the Internet, this viral would not have been as far reaching, and not have resulted in her leaving university, humiliated (Solove, 2007). The Internet, arguably, has made such incidents far more common and much easier for the everyday person to partake in. Crucially, many people are also complicit in this erosion of privacy, in particular through the use of SNS to share personal information with peers and marketing organizations.

PRIVACY OF SOCIAL NETWORKING SITES

Typically, privacy concerns online have related to e-commerce transactions, notably credit card fraud, vendors' use of personal details, and customer identification (Miyazaki & Fernandez, 2000), but with growing concern over what users are posting online, the concern is no longer related solely to such issues. In relation to SNS, this tends to develop around the topic of identity fraud based on users' posting of information on their profiles or the SNS itself allowing unrestricted "default" access (e.g., Acquisti & Gross, 2009; Gross & Acquisti, 2005; Lampe, Ellison, & Steinfield, 2007; Young & Quan-Haase, 2009). Although identity fraud, credit card fraud, and data storage concerns are undoubtedly alarming, privacy is also harmed by users' own behavior, such as teenagers' trend of "sexting" one another (Betts, 2009), cyberbullying (Reed, 2009), and the inability to control one's social spheres on SNS (Binder et al., 2009).

Privacy can be viewed from the perspective of control. Whether it is control over personal data, the choice to disclose data, the physical presence of others, the number of others present in disclosure, or choosing which person to discuss and share issues with, control is central to maintaining privacy (e.g., Altman, 1975; DeCew, 1997; Solove, 2006; Warren & Brandeis, 1890). In particular, Altman, with his emphasis on social interaction with our environment, proposed the concept of personal, dyadic, and group boundaries for controlling privacy and disclosure (Altman, 1975). In daily off line life, these boundaries tend to be obvious. We are aware of who we are talking to, through vocalization or bodily posture and gestures; who we write to; what we have heard and from whom; who can see us walk down the street; who can see us use the toilet; if cameras are pointed at us (although some closed-circuit television requires actively looking for it); who or what has touched us; and who and what we have touched (whether friendly or unfriendly). However, controlling these boundaries and the information flow between them in a SNS environment can prove difficult due to the eclectic use of the term "friend" (Binder et al., 2009). In an SNS, the term "friend" is often used to denote any number of potential relationship ties.

TYPES OF RELATIONSHIP TIE

The need to control the flow of personal information to different types of relationship tie is central to our social world. We allow certain more detailed, intimate aspects of ourselves to be released or shared with another as part of a private bond of intimacy, whereas we release less information to those who we to hold a lesser intimate relationship with (Rachels, 1975; Reiman, 1976). For example, we may share different information with an intimate partner than with a parent. Reiman (1976) notes, "Only because we are able to withhold personal information about—and forbid intimate observation of—ourselves from the rest of the world, can we give out personal information—and allow intimate observations—to friends and/or lovers, that constitute intimate relationships" (p. 31).

In deciding which elements of one's personality and personal information to release to various types of relationship, the centrality of each may be useful in determining how intimate or detailed the information is. Altman and Taylor (1973) describe the centrality of personality as similar to different and deepening layers of an onion. The centrality of individuals within a social network has been suggested to relate to levels of expected privacy. If personal information is taken by another and spread to connections further from the individual than would reasonably be expected by their own means and intimate friend group then it is argued as a violation of privacy (Strahilivetz, 2004).

In online interaction, such as a SNS, the distinction between who is able to see, obtain, and use various bits of our data or image becomes blurred. Virtuality creates a person management problem (Handy, 1995). By adding multiple types of "ties" to our "friends" list on, for example, Facebook, it becomes difficult to manage access and sharing with different people and types of "friend" (Binder et al., 2009; DiMicco & Millen, 2007). For example, photos of drunken excursions may be willingly shared with friends, but are they so eagerly shared with family, work colleagues, or even potential employers? Online, unless controlled and managed through often complicated privacy settings, everybody in the "friends" list can access these photos. Therefore, managing social spheres becomes complicated (Binder et al., 2009; DiMicco & Millen, 2007), and such complications and unforeseen circumstances may lead to privacy harms.

Issues of privacy on SNS can depend on the site used and the user's site settings and personal privacy preferences. For instance, Facebook provides the ability to create a visible personal profile including photographs, hometown, date of birth, relationship status, and e-mail address (e.g., Christofides, Muise, & Desmarais, 2009; Joinson, 2008; Lampe et al., 2007) that is then openly available to potentially unknown others. Furthermore, unless privacy settings are customized, users may be unaware to whom they are disseminating information. Release of personal and private information may cause additional security problems including phishing, information leakage, and stalking (Gross & Acquisti, 2005; Hasib, 2008; Westlake, 2008). Social network sites that do not openly provide personal details are not exempt from privacy issues, potentially providing enough information to identify the user, such as by a photograph common with other SNS by default (Gross & Acquisti, 2005). Recent changes to the privacy settings of Facebook have further complicated this issue by making much information (e.g., photographs, lists of "friends") open to everyone by default for the majority of users.

Discussion of privacy and social network sites has tended to focus on the potential threat posed by either outside access, such as reidentifying profile pictures, demographic data, or unique interests from other SNS (Gross & Acquisti, 2005). Other outside threats may originate in the general use of unsecured login connections used by SNS allowing easy access for third parties, such as hackers, identity thieves, and government (Gross & Acquisti, 2005). However, there are further privacy issues within the SNS and the network of contacts, even if private information is willingly disclosed by a site user (Gross & Acquisti, 2005). These include the open discussion of personal information among contacts, the posting and tagging of photographs that identify other users, disclosure of demographic data, and posting personal information on profile pages that implicates other users (Acquisti & Gross, 2006; Christofides et al., 2009). Furthermore, the availability of hometown and date of birth information has been shown to facilitate the calculation of Social Security numbers (SSN) in the United States (Acquisti & Gross, 2009).

Bonneau and Preibusch (2009) report a wide variety in the privacy control settings available across the 45 SNS they visited. Bonneau and Preibusch (2009) add that privacy policies, privacy controls, and informative measures are often complicated and below expectancy. In managing privacy within a SNS, sites rarely publicize their privacy enhancing tools even if they are available (Bonneau & Preibusch, 2009). Thus, if users are unaware that privacy threats exist, they are not likely to be prompted by the SNS that does not publicize such features, and so the unknown information sharing may continue. SNS may not publicize their features due to the effects of privacy salience: even for unconcerned users, raising attention to privacy controls may lead to users becoming more cautious and to sharing less information (Bonneau

& Preibusch, 2009), perhaps reducing the richness of content and thus user experience and contribution (Burke, Marlow, & Lento, 2009).

Privacy concerns are rife throughout modern Internet usage. The increasing number of SNS and SNS users makes information sharing and concealing difficult to manage. The cumulative nature of social spheres, or relationship types, under the "friends" umbrella in SNS works only to amplify the issues. Users are often unaware of ubiquitous and large scale data collection and storage (Sparck Jones, 2003) and are often unaware of the harms of a collective "friends" group (Binder et al., 2009). Frequently researched privacy issues of online and SNS use typically include credit card fraud, identity theft, and what type of information users put on their SNS profiles (Acquisti & Gross, 2009). Although such issues are concerning, it is not clear what participants deem to be privacy violations or if their concerns match those of researchers.

To determine the difficulties and consequences of managing and experiencing a privacy violation, we interviewed a number of participants about their experiences and friendships. Although we asked about privacy violations in general rather than online, it became apparent that a majority of interviewees experienced a privacy violation due to their use of Facebook. Furthermore, as privacy can be seen as a control mechanism for limiting certain information flows to different types of relationship tie, we asked interviewees what friends and friendship meant to them to explore such links with privacy.

METHODOLOGY

This exploratory study used an open and unstructured approach to enhance the understanding and knowledge of what people mean when discussing friendships, privacy, and privacy violations. An opportunistic sample of eight individuals were interviewed using an unstructured approach but were provided with an initial question and discussion to set the topic. The 8 individuals were aged between 23 and 32 years old, of whom 3 were male and 5 were female. All participants had an education of at least an undergraduate degree, but from different disciplines. Participants were interviewed in similar, quiet environments at their convenience. The interviews were recorded using open source software (Audacity) and a standard PC microphone, and each lasted approximately 15 minutes, ranging from 10–26 minutes. Care was taken by the interviewer to avoid the use of leading questions or suggestive body language to ensure that the participant felt comfortable, open to discussion, and unbiased.

Participants were initially asked what their friendships meant to them followed by questions about a privacy violation that they had experienced at some point in their lives. This was to allow an insight into the results of privacy violations on friendships before and after a violation had occurred. Friendships and their benefits were asked about in general terms, whereas the questioning related to the privacy violation was more specific.

Ethical concerns, while only marginal, were considered, thus steps were taken to reduce such risk. Informed consent was given. Participants were told of their right to withdraw their data at any point. Participants were informed that they could give as much or as little detail as they felt comfortable with and were reminded of this during the interview when privacy issues were discussed. The interviewer was not to coerce further information from the interviewee if the topic seemed potentially upsetting or too sensitive. Finally, should any unforeseen consequences have arisen, the interviewee could discuss these with the interviewer, who could then advise on suitable help and referral to specialists in that area (using the NHS Direct Web site).

Of the eight participants, all the interviews were transcribed, and none indicated any distress or wish to withdraw their data from this study. Thematic analyses were then conducted on the transcriptions to reveal modal themes and issues.

RESULTS AND DISCUSSION

The interviews highlighted a variety of issues relating to what friendship meant to each participant and what constituted a privacy violation. Some interviewees were relatively certain in their conceptualization of privacy, whereas others were more unsure. Privacy violations were varied, too. Some participants were unable to recall a privacy violation or were unconcerned that their privacy could be violated, whereas others were more certain about what had happened and what it meant to maintain privacy.

Of the eight privacy violations discussed by participants, five related specifically to social network sites, and three to off line violations (although they incorporated technology in some form or other). The violations reported are outlined in Table 1.

Common Issues with Violations

Participants' usual response on experiencing, or becoming aware of, a privacy violation was to change their relationship with the violator, on one occasion even when the violator was clearly an innocent bystander. P5, for example, was subject to a third party using a friend's Facebook account in an attempt to elicit money from her via a cry for help using the chat feature. Acknowledging that this was a loose friend, the participant transferred some of the blame onto the friend and has not spoken to the friend since.

TABLE 1 Summary of Privacy Violations Reported by Participants

Participant	Summary of violation
P1	Boyfriend sharing detailed relationship information with a friend via the public medium of the Facebook "wall" feature
P2	A confidant sharing sensitive financial information (failures) with a group of mutual friends
P3	Postal service employee obtaining credit cards and the personal information needed to activate them then using them to purchase valuable items
P4	A trusted friend dropping subtle comments into a conversation with a group of friends that could potentially allow this entrusted, dyadic information to become group knowledge
P5	An unauthorized user of an acquaintance's Facebook account attempting to persuade the participant to transfer large sums of money to their account using the Facebook "chat" (instant messaging) feature
P6	A (now ex-) boyfriend discussed snide comments the participant had made with their parents, leading them to think she was not a good or appropriate person or girlfriend
P7	Friends using a Facebook group discussion board to gossip about silly things from the participant's past, issues she no longer wishes to discuss or have discussed about her
P8	Discusses several issues to do with Facebook friends but focuses on an off line violation—the participant's mother went through his room and discovered a home pregnancy test kit and discussed it with one of the participant's friends, who in turn used it to mock the participant, leading him to feel annoyed with his mother for (a) snooping in his room and (b) sharing the information with others

Furthermore, P5 has "defriended" the person on Facebook with no further contact (Facebook being their only means to communicate).

Incurring an emotional or surprised response to a violation appeared unanimous across all interviews. Participants commented on feeling "upset," "angry," and "shocked." For example, P1, who had recently broken up with her partner, suffered a privacy violation because this partner put details of the relationship's demise onto a mutual friend's Facebook wall. This led the participant to be "so shocked that he would do that, because it was sort of unfeeling . . . not cruel but . . . harsh." When discussing this further the participant suggested that timing was key to the "painful experience . . . of [it] broadcast everywhere." P1 noted that because the violation had occurred approximately two days after the breakup of the relationship (perceived as a short time by P1, especially for a three-year relationship), it may have caused more harm, suggesting that "if it had been later on, I don't think it would've annoyed me."

Across the interviews, time was frequently mentioned in reactions to privacy violations. Time was a concern if too brief a period passed between discussing something with another and their subsequent dissemination of the information, as in the case of P1, P2, P4, and P6 (see Table 1). Time was also a concern when a violation occurred too close to the sensitive event, such as

P1, P2, P4, and P8 (see Table 1). In addition, P8 alluded to being caught "preparing to masturbate on my bed" and feeling "a little bit embarrassed" but that "ten minutes later, I went outside, faced the music, people laughed at me, I got over it." P8 demonstrates that even if rather brief, there was an initial shock in the information dissemination quite soon after the event. Time was discussed further in reference to looking back at the violation after a long period and consequently no longer finding it harmful or painful. For instance, P6 said that "now the relationship's over it doesn't really matter, they [sic] can tell them all they want for all I care."

Furthermore, participants were concerned with the ways in which friends/trusted others did not behave in the manner in which they expected a trusted other to behave with regard to their information. For example, P1 was "shocked" that her partner would divulge information about their relationship publicly. Also, participants found the friendship itself to be misinterpreted, resulting in a behavior that was unexpected at the time but would perhaps have been expected if they knew what sort of relationship they shared with the other person. For example, P2 said, "To me, it was really out of line...she didn't realise what was wrong...and the understanding...that I could just tell her things that are on my mind [was not there]." Uncertainty Reduction Theory (URT) argues that people are motivated to reduce uncertainty in relationships, in particular about the character of the other person or their commitment and beliefs (Berger & Calabrese, 1975). To reduce uncertainty, we need to trade information with the people with whom we communicate (Berger & Calabrese, 1975). Therefore, to understand the expectancies of the dyad, individuals should share information to reduce uncertainty in their future behaviors before sharing more detailed personal information. Furthermore, Berger (1979) suggests three preconditions for uncertainty reduction: deviations from expected behavior, potential costs or rewards, and the likelihood of future interaction. A misunderstanding of these, similar to a misunderstanding due to poorly negotiated rules in communication privacy management (Petronio, 2002), may explain why participants endured a privacy violation and found it unpleasant emotionally. In the previous examples, the experienced unpleasantness was the participant's surprise of the trusted other's deviation from behavioral expectancy and the trusted other's inability to realize the detrimental impact on their future interactions.

Many of the issues discussed previously are similar to issues raised by Petronio (2002) in her theory of communication privacy management (CPM). When participants' expectations of others' behavior differs from actual behavior, the implicit rule negotiation is broken and the management of information has failed. In sharing information with another or via an SNS, the participants were unaware of the condition of the boundaries surrounding them and their information. "Condition" refers to the permeability of the boundary and the choice of the trusted other to respect it or break it if it prevented their sharing of this information. In online communication, sharing information with new contacts may serve to reduce uncertainty of their behavior and intentions (Tidwell & Walther, 2002), but this may also lead to increased risk of privacy management issues. Thus, boundary control becomes erroneous, highlighting the difficulties of maintaining multiple social spheres, as noted by Binder and colleagues (2009) and DiMicco and Millen (2007).

CPM also defines information as co-owned once shared. Participants expecting the information to be entirely controlled by themselves may not have appreciated the idea that once information is shared, the recipient becomes a co-owner (Petronio, 2002), and while the desire of the sharer should be respected, it often may not be. For example, P6 was concerned that "my boyfriend would go away and tell his parents" about arguments that had arisen in their relationship. This is contrary to the view taken in the late 19th century by Warren and Brandeis (1890) that information should remain the right of the creator, and subsequently even letters written to others should remain in control of the author. Only when writings are published do they suggest that ownership is relinquished.

Today, in a ubiquitous computing environment with users creating much of the content of Web 2.0, it is increasingly important for users to realize the nature of boundaries, possible violations, and the importance of ownership of information. While it is not wholly acceptable to generalize from such a small sample, the participants of this sample population illustrate a few of the difficulties in establishing and maintaining operational privacy boundaries in the online ubiquitous society of today.

Thematic Analysis

From the range of privacy issues discussed in the interviews, a thematic analysis was conducted to determine several broader categories based on participants' responses and information divulged. Items were first split by whether they represented either friendship in general or a privacy violation. The data in each split were then ranked by the total number of utterances a particular category received across all interviews. Data that arose from three or more utterances were filtered by the number of participants that uttered them. Any themes uttered less than thrice were removed to ensure the utterance constituted a repetitive theme. This resulted in 18 categories for privacy violations and 16 categories for general friendship components (see Tables 2 and 3, respectively).

This thematic analysis on privacy violations surfaces four main issues underlying the majority of mentioned themes: issues of control, boundary expectations and uncertainties, an initial shock/startle reaction, and a temporal component whereby the situation may be perceived differently. The privacy themes suggest a basis in Uncertainty Reduction Theory.

TABLE 2 Thematic Analysis of Privacy Violations: Recurring Themes and the Number of Occurrences Across All Interviews

Category/Theme	Frequency
Uncertainty of information spread (loss of control)	11
Time component	8
Upsetting emotional reaction	8
Disparity of boundary rules	7
Release/share information outside of dyad/relationship	7
Increased caution/awareness (specific)	7
Expectancy to maintain boundary/secret	6
Shock/surprised emotional reaction	5
Increased caution/awareness (general)	5
Too many others know (or shared with)	4
Defriended	4
No value to violator (or loss)	4
Separation of violator from his or her org./group	4
Angry emotional reaction	3
Disparity/conflict of trust (loss of trust included)	3
No value to victim (or loss)	3
Not talk in public with others	3
Feeling embarrassed	3

In particular, initial interactions are suggested to be a key time period whereby communication is increased to reduce uncertainty (Berger & Calabrese, 1975), and it is in initial dissemination of new information whereby privacy harms are most sensitive, suggested by a shock/startle reaction.

TABLE 3 Thematic Analysis of the Concept of Friendship: Recurring Themes and the Number of Occurrences Across All Interviews

Category/Theme	Frequency
Different types of friends (e.g., some to socialize, some for humor, some to feel secure, some due to proximity)	18
Common experiences or tastes	12
Trust (inc. reciprocal trust and varying degrees of)	10
Sharing (non-descript)	9
To share humor/amusement	6
Feeling secure (security)	6
Count on/rely on/fall back on	6
Being close	6
To socialize	5
Respect	5
Reciprocal (e.g., giving and taking)	5
Enjoyment	4
Solve issues (gain inspiration)	3
Ask for help	3
Friends reflect part of you	3
Geographically unconcerned (far but close, close but far)	3

Issues of Control

Issues of control typically related to the participant feeling they had no or little control over the occurrence of a privacy violation. P1 was upset that the dissemination of the information was unsure and out of her immediate control: "It came up on the news feeds. . . . I don't know [if] everybody gets the same news feeds but it came up on the news feeds." P1 adds, "There wasn't anything I could really do about it because . . . you can't go onto somebody else's wall and delete it." Control issues arose for P3 when he felt "quite sick because I didn't know what to do." P5 discussed readjusting privacy settings on Facebook after a privacy violation to gain control over the access others have to her information. P5 also defriended their friend's Facebook account to prevent future occurrences or an immediate risk of data leakage to the unauthorized third party. P6 discussed control in terms of wanting to "make a good impression on [her boyfriend's] parents" and that issues arose when she could not control her boyfriend from "go[ing] to their [sic] parents and say 'she's done this and she's done that.'" When P7 discovered widespread dissemination of gossip about her as a child she removed herself from that Facebook group and would speak to the members only individually.

Control as a method to manage privacy is suggested by privacy theorists and finds support in these interviews. For example, "Selective control of access to the self" (Altman, 1975, p. 24) and "the claim of individuals, groups, or institutions to determine for themselves when, how and to what extent information about them is communicated to others" (Westin, 1967, p. 7). Furthermore, in Petronio's (2002) theory of CPM she notes that boundaries can be used as a mechanism of control and are instigated by rule negotiation. Such boundaries are protected from loss of control by the enforcement of consequences, such as ex-communication. Support is found here from P2 who says that "we are not friends anymore."

Boundary Expectancies and Uncertainties

The second underlying issue is how participants have an expectation of a boundary of privacy. A violation then occurs when the boundary is broken, either deliberately or unintentionally. Work on boundaries for maintaining privacy was proposed as a method of controlling physical access to the self or access to the intimate zone surrounding an individual (Altman, 1975). Furthermore, by instigating these physical boundaries it allows a physical and mental environment for one to reflect and self-evaluate (Altman, 1975; Westin, 1967). This issue is taken further to include boundaries for withholding information about the self and the co-ownership of such information when it is shared within such boundaries (Altman, 1975; Petronio, 2002). Support for idea of boundary usage in information management is found in URT. Managing communication boundaries and sharing information is motivated by a need to reduce uncertainty of others (Berger, 1979).

Such boundary issues and motivations are raised by the interviewees when discussing privacy violations. P1 says that her partner shared "a lot of information...more than I would have expected him to mention." P2 experienced a disrupted dyadic boundary when "[name] just turned around and told everyone." P4 became aware of the need to manage her boundaries in future because her friend "may not keep things to herself, and [because of] her judgement of what is something for her or something that she could say to everyone else." P8 suffered an issue of boundary disparity when his mother broke the dyadic boundary around himself and his girlfriend by snooping around his room and finding a pregnancy test kit.

As noted earlier, controlling such differing social spheres becomes difficult on SNS because they are often converged to a single tie type (Binder et al., 2009; DiMicco & Millen, 2007; Gilbert & Karahalios, 2009). P1's privacy violation broke the dyadic boundary surrounding her and her partner to all those that had access to a mutual friend's Facebook wall. Those with access could be friends, family, or colleagues of one or multiple of the three parties. P7 endured privacy harms when stories and gossip from primary school were spread around a group of friends that she now had little or nothing in common with. Ideally, the information would have stayed between the very few who knew or alternatively have been discussed only by those with whom she is close. In this instance, the converging spheres were different types of friends rather than a friend and a family sphere blurring.

Initial Startle/Shock Reaction

The interview data suggests that the majority of participants' initial reaction to a privacy violation was either to be shocked/startled or to have an emotional reaction such as anger or upset. This concept was closely related to that of "time" in the temporal component, as participants frequently mentioned being shocked at how soon the information had been disseminated. Alternatively, the shock resulted in others discussing events that occurred too far in the past. For example, P7 reacted to information about her becoming public on Facebook by saying that "for me it's [a] bit annoying because I don't want someone [to] actually talk about me in public and they even post lots of photos of me when I was a kid." P1 reported, "It was just a shock for me when I first saw it." P2 said, "I honestly wasn't expecting her to just go around and tell everyone I know.... How could she have done that to me?" P3 reflected, "I was very shocked. I then felt quite sick." P4 agreed with the interviewer that there was a shock reaction to the violation. P6 admitted to feeling "a bit angry" about her boyfriend's open discussion of private matters with his parents. P8 recalled being "really quite angry" at his mother and even "confronted her about it" and "also quite angry towards her friend for bringing it up" when discussing the violation regarding his mother's covert discovery of a pregnancy test kit.

Contrary to the deficit of such immediacy of information, SNS such as Facebook typically encourage interaction based on current thoughts, links, events, and discussions. For example, when posting a new status update, sharing a link or sharing a photograph on Facebook, the text box asks "What's on your mind?" Answering in this immediate time frame may encourage users to post information before giving thorough thought to potential consequences. Such behavior may subsequently result in privacy harms and violations for themselves and others.

Time and a Temporal Component

This last underlying category demonstrates the temporal nature of privacy, that time can be not only a healer but that a lack of time can agitate the immediacy of the unpleasant emotion. Time, then, is a fundamental privacy process. Privacy preferences are said to be different for different situations, contexts, and points in time, and desired privacy fluctuates over time (Altman, 1975; DeCew, 1997; Petronio, 2002; Westin, 2003). The data from these interviews supports this notion yet further identifies that privacy violations do not necessarily result in defriending. Forgiveness may occur when such trust is breached within online interaction, as is suggested by Vasalou, Hopfensitz, and Pitt (2008).

P1 reflected a change in the anger she felt at the time and at the present: "Not now, but at the time." P2, however, is no longer a friend with the violator once the "trust . . . and respect" had gone. P3's insight is optimistic of a "worst case scenario" whereby a friend created a serious breach of trust but reflects on the idea that a true friend would have such a deep trust that any privacy violation would be repairable and perhaps would even strengthen the relationship.

Friendship Aspects

DIFFERENT TYPES OF FRIEND (TIE)

The most common theme throughout the interviews for friendship was that there are different types of friend. Participants spoke of the different things they enjoy with some friends and the implicit links between the type of friend and the expectancies associated with it. For example, P2 suggested that friends could be there to have fun with or to be a "safety net." This links closely with work on management of boundaries. Boundaries are suggested to allow an individual (or group) to control who has access to different information about them and to determine when and in what situations this information is transferred (Altman, 1975; Petronio, 2002). Additionally, different types of "tie," or friend, exist within a social network, both off line and online. Ties are suggested to vary based on network structure and their position within the network (Granovetter, 1973; Haythornthwaite, 1996).

Rachels (1975) and Reiman (1976) both propose that we share more information about ourselves with those with whom we wish to be intimate to allow a social distinction of the type of relationship had. Therefore, we can determine that if a friend we thought of as particularly close does not share the same detailed information in return, this friend may not consider himself or herself as close a friend as we do him or her (Rachels, 1975; Reiman, 1976). In SNS contexts, ties are usually compounded as only one type, although this has caused discussion in the difficulties of managing the boundaries surrounding the realistic and actual occurrence of multiple tie types (Binder et al., 2009; DiMicco & Millen, 2007).

In our interviews, P3 discusses having different types of friend for different purpose. He suggests that friends who are proximally close are not necessarily those whom he considers his closest friends. His closest friends are those whom he has known since childhood despite their geographic dispersion. About longstanding friends, he says they are "the type of friends where the friendship is based on trust." Whereas regarding his local friends he suggests they are "perhaps valuable in the sense of a career or contacts."

Trust

The topic of trust was mentioned frequently across all interviews. CPM theory suggests that with those with whom we share personal information, there is a requirement that the shared boundary is thick, or less permeable. We expect information to be kept within the boundary due to trust in implicit or negotiated rules that the other parties are expected to sustain.

When discussing friendships, a number of participants suggested that trust is a very important factor. For example, P2 said, "I think trust is important between two people, if they want to share information, and also with trust that comes openness and respect." This quote also highlights the importance of reciprocity in relationships.

Reciprocal Interaction

The topic of reciprocal interaction includes the categories of *common experiences or tastes, sharing* (nondescript), and any utterances that discussed a *reciprocal* interaction. P3 discusses that friends are people "who make the effort back . . . and they incite me to do in return." Furthermore, he mentions that some friendships are based on "common interests, it's social interaction, we go out, we do things together that we both like doing." P4 indicates that friendship is about "sharing something with you." P5 alludes to having "friendships because you have things in common with those people... people you work with or live with or go to uni with."

Support for the nature of sharing common items as a method to reduce cohesion and build relationships can be found in social psychology literature on group conflict (e.g., Eisenhardt, Kahwajy, & Bourgeois III, 1997; Sherif, 1958). Furthermore, the reduction of individual differences for success has been investigated within online global virtual teams that use ICTs (Panteli & Sockalingam, 2005).

CONCLUSIONS

This work aimed to determine what happens before and after a privacy violation with regard to friendship and resultant relationship changes. The data developed through a series of open interviews on what privacy and friendship meant to the participants and on their examples and thoughts about experienced violations. Although there are many and countering theories, circumstances, dynamic demands, and subjective and objective approaches to privacy, it is important to determine that what is theorized is what is experienced. The interviews have shown and supported many of the aspects of privacy as shown in the discussion. However, it is acknowledged that there are numerous other issues surrounding privacy, what has become apparent are the key concepts from this sample.

The sample supports the idea of boundaries within which information can be shared, the importance of co-owned information, that different boundaries exist around different types of friend or tie, and that privacy issues are ubiquitous with online SNS use. Furthermore, with such large scale use and development of SNS in the culture of the Internet, managing these boundaries, social spheres, aspects of information, and the relationships they entail may become increasingly difficult. It is necessary for users to be aware of such issues before they are experienced and for the development of SNS to include the options to prioritize information with different social spheres, similar to that managed physically in off-line environments. Currently, Facebook and LinkedIn are the only SNS to allow users to view their profile from the perspective of other users to see what information is visible about them (Bonneau & Preibusch, 2009).

Limitations

Although this work embraces the subjectivity of the qualitative, open methodology used, there are several limitations that are acknowledged here. The small sample size will affect the ability to generalize this sample to the greater population. There are also a number of topics that were raised in the interviews that were unfortunately not discussed within this article due to scope limitations. However, this work can be used as an indication and building block as to what are seen as important aspects of privacy to those not knowledgeable of or researching the area.

REFERENCES

Acquisti, A., & Gross, R. (2006). Imagined communities: Awareness, information sharing, and privacy on Facebook. Paper presented at the Privacy Enhancing Technology workshop. Cambridge, UK, June 28–June 30.

Acquisti, A., & Gross, R. (2009). Social insecurity: The unintended consequences of identity fraud prevention policies. Paper presented at the Workshop on the Economics of Information Security, University College London.

Altman, I. (1975). *The environment and social behavior*. Belmont, CA: Wadsworth.

Altman, I., & Taylor, D. A. (1973). *Social penetration: The development of interpersonal relationships*. Austin, TX: Holt, Rinehart and Winston.

Anawati, D., & Craig, A. (2006). Behavioral adaptation within cross-cultural virtual teams. *IEEE transactions on professional communication, 49*(1), 44–56.

Berger, C. R. (1979). Beyond initial interaction: Uncertainty, understanding, and the development of interpersonal relationships. In H. Giles & R. St. Clair (Eds.), *Language and social psychology*, (pp. 122–144). Oxford: Blackwell.

Berger, C. R., & Calabrese, R. J. (1975). Some explorations in initial interaction and beyond: Toward a developmental theory of interpersonal communication. *Human communication research, 1*, 99–112.

Betts, H. (2009, October). Generation reveal: There's nothing they won't post online. *TimesOnline*. Retrieved from http://women.timesonline.co.uk/tol/life_and_style/women/relationships/article6861770.ece.

Binder, J., Howes, A., & Sutcliffe, A. (2009). The problem of conflicting social spheres: Effects of network structure on experienced tension in social network sites. Paper presented at Computer Human Interaction 2009, Boston, Massachusetts.

Bonneau, J., & Preibusch, S. (2009). The privacy jungle: On the market for data protection in social networks. Paper presented at the Workshop on the Economics of Information Security, University College London.

Boyd, D. M., & Ellison, N. B. (2007). Social network sites: Definition, history and scholarship. *Journal of Computer-Mediated Communication, 13*(1), 210–230.

Burgoon, J. K., Parrott, R., le Poire, B. A., & Kelley, D. L. (1989). Maintaining and restoring privacy through communication in different types of relationships. *Journal of Social and Personal Relationships, 6*(2), 131–158.

Burke, M., Marlow, C., & Lento, T. (2009). Feed me: Motivating newcomer contribution in social network sites. Paper presented at Computer Human Interaction 2009, Boston, Massachusetts.

Christofides, E., Muise, A., & Desmarais, S. (2009). Information disclosure and control on Facebook: Are they two sides of the same coin or two different processes? *CyberPsychology & Behavior, 12*(3), 341–345.

DeCew, J. W. (1997). *In pursuit of privacy: Law, ethics, and the rise of technology*. Ithaca, NY: Cornell University Press.

DiMicco, J. M., & Millen, D. R. (2007). Identity management: Multiple presentations of self in Facebook. Paper presented at the Proceedings of the 2007 International Association for Computing Machinery conference on Supporting Groupwork, Sanibel Island, Florida.

Eisenhardt, K. M., Kahwajy, J. L., & Bourgeois III, L. J. (1997). How management teams can have a good fight. *Harvard Business Review, 75*(4), 77–85.

Ellison, N., Steinfeld, C., & Lampe, C. (2007). The benefits of Facebook "friends": Exploring the relationship between college students' use of online social networks and social capital. *Journal of Computer-Mediated Communication, 12*(3), 1143–1168.

Facebook. (2010). Press room: Statistics. Retrieved from: http://www.facebook.com/press/info.php?statistics

"Facebook remark teenager is fired." (2009). BBC News. Retrieved from http://news.bbc.co.uk/1/hi/england/essex/7914415.stm

Gilbert, E., & Karahalios, K. (2009). Predicting tie strength with social Media. Paper presented at Computer Human Interaction 2009, Boston, Massachusetts.

Golder, S., Wilkinson, D., & Huberman, B. (2007). Rhythms of social interaction: Messaging within a massive online network. In *Third international conference on communities and technologies* (pp. 41–66). London, UK: Springer.

Granovetter, M. S. (1973). The strength of weak ties. *The American Journal of Sociology, 78*(6), 1360.

Gross, R., & Acquisti, A. (2005). Information revelation and privacy in online social networks. Paper presented at the Proceedings of the 2005 Association for Computing Machinery workshop on Privacy in the Electronic Society, Alexandria, Virginia.

Handy, C. (1995). Trust and the virtual organization. *Harvard Business Review, 73*(3), 40–50.

Hasebrink, U., Livingstone, S., Haddon, L., & Ólafsson, K. (Eds.). (2009). *Comparing children's online opportunities and risks across Europe: Cross-national comparisons for EU Kids Online*, (2nd ed.). LSE, London: EU Kids Online.

Hasib, A. A. (2008). *Threats of online social networks*. Helsinki, Finland: Helsinki University of Technology.

Haythornthwaite, C. (1996). Social network analysis: An approach and technique for the study of information exchange. *Library & Information Science Research, 18*(4), 323–342.

Joinson, A. N. (2008). "Looking at," "looking up" or "keeping up with" people? Motives and uses of Facebook. Paper presented at the CHI Helsinki, Finland 2008—Online Social Networks, Florence, Italy.

Joinson, A. N. (2009). *Privacy concerns, trust in government and attitudes to identity cards in the United Kingdom*. Unpublished manuscript.

Jones, S. G. (Ed.). (1995). *CyberSociety: Computer-mediated communication and community*. SAGE Publications.

Kraut, R., Kiesler, S., Boneva, B., Cummings, J. N., Helgeson, V., & Crawford, A. M. (2002). Internet paradox revisited. *Journal of Social Issues, 58*(1), 49–74.

Kraut, R., Patterson, M., Lundmark, V., Kiesler, S., Mukophadhyay, T., & Scherlis, W. (1998). Internet paradox: A social technology that reduces social involvement and psychological well-being? *American Psychologist, 53*(9), 10171–10031.

Krueger, B. S. (2005). Government surveillance and political participation on the Internet. *Social Science Computer Review, 23*(4), 439.

Lampe, C., Ellison, N., & Steinfield, C. (2006). A face(book) in the crowd: Social searching vs. social browsing. Paper presented at the Proceedings of the 2006 20th anniversary conference on Computer Supported Cooperative Work, Banff, Alberta, Canada.

Lampe, C., Ellison, N., & Steinfield, C. (2007). A familiar face(book): Profile elements as signals in an online social network. Paper presented at the Proceedings of the Special Interest Group on Computer Human Interaction conference on Human factors in computing systems, San Jose, California.

Lipsman, A. (2010). 2009: Another strong year for Facebook. Retrieved from http://blog.comscore.com/2010/01/strong_year_for_facebook.html

Margulis, S. T. (2003). On the status and contribution of Westin's and Altman's theories of privacy. *The Journal of Social Issues, 59*(2), 411–429.

Miyazaki, A. D., & Fernandez, A. (2000). Internet privacy and security: An examination of online retailer disclosures. *Journal of Public Policy & Marketing, 19*(1), 54–61.

Panteli, N., & Sockalingam, S. (2005). Trust and conflict within virtual inter-organizational alliances: A framework for facilitating knowledge sharing. *Decision Support Systems, 39*(4), 599.

Parent, W. A. (1983). Privacy, morality, and the law. *Philosophy and Public Affairs, 12*(4), 269–288.

Petronio, S. (2002). *Boundaries of privacy*. Albany: State University of New York.

Rachels, J. (1975). Why privacy is important. *Philosophy and Public Affairs, 4*(4), 323–333.

Reed, J. (2009, November). Facebook "bully" explains actions. BBC News. Retrieved from http://news.bbc.co.uk/newsbeat/hi/front_page/newsid_10000000/newsid_10002900/10002995.stm

Reiman, J. H. (1976). Privacy, intimacy, and personhood. *Philosophy and Public Affairs, 6*(1), 26–44.

Schatz Byford, K. (1996). Privacy in cyberspace: Constructing a model of privacy for the electronic communications environment. *Rutgers Computer and Technology Law Journal, 24*, 1–74.

Schoeman, F. D. (1984). *Philosophical dimensions of privacy: An anthology*. Cambridge, UK: Cambridge University Press.

Sherif, M. (1958). Superordinate goals in the reduction of intergroup conflict. *The American Journal of Sociology, LXIII*(4), 349–356.

Solove, D. J. (2006). A taxonomy of privacy. *University of Pennsylvania Law Review, 154*(3), 477.

Solove, D. J. (2007). *The future of reputation: Gossip, rumor, and privacy on the Internet*. New Haven: Yale University Press.

Sparck Jones, K. (2003). Privacy: What's different now? *Interdisciplinary Science Reviews, 28*(4), 287–292.

Strahilivetz, L. J. (2004). A social networks theory of privacy. John M. Olin Law & Economics Working Paper No. 230. The Law School, University of Chicago.

Tidwell, L. C., & Walther, J. B. (2002). Computer-mediated communication effects on disclosure, impressions, and interpersonal evaluations: Getting to know one another a bit at a time. *Human Communication Research, 28*(3), 317–348.

UK Office of National Statistics. (2008, August). Internet access 2008: Households and individuals. Retrieved from http://www.statistics.gov.uk/pdfdir/iahi0808.pdf

Vasalou, A., Hopfensitz, A., & Pitt, J. (2008). In praise of forgiveness: Ways for repairing trust breakdowns in one-off online interactions. *International Journal of Human–Computer Studies*, *66*(6), 466–480.

Warren, S. V., & Brandeis, L. D. (1890). The right to privacy. *Harvard Law Review*, *4*(5), 193–220.

Westin, A. F. (1967). *Privacy and freedom*. New York: Athenaeum.

Westin, A. F. (2003). Social and political dimensions of privacy. *Journal of Social Issues*, *59*(2), 431–453.

Westlake, E. J. (2008). Friend me if you Facebook: Generation Y and performative surveillance. *The Drama Review*, *52*(4), 21.

Young, A. L., & Quan-Haase, A. (2009). Information revelation and Internet privacy concerns on social network sites: A case study of Facebook. Paper presented at Communities and Technologies '09, University Park, Pennsylvania.

Corporate Parenting in the Network Society

NEIL BALLANTYNE

Glasgow School of Social Work, University of Strathclyde, Glasgow, United Kingdom

ZACHARI DUNCALF

Scottish Institute for Residential Child Care, University of Strathclyde, Glasgow, United Kingdom

ELLEN DALY

Institute for Research and Innovation in Social Services, Glasgow, United Kingdom

In the past few years the risks associated with use of the Internet and social networking sites by children and young people have become a recurrent focus of attention for the media, the public, and policymakers. Parents, caregivers, and child care professionals alike are rightly concerned about exposure to pornography, pedophiles, and cyberbullies. At the same time Internet researchers have been steadily collecting evidence about the actual opportunities and risks associated with the young people's use of the Internet. In this article we describe some of the emerging evidence on opportunities and risks for young people and consider the challenges for social welfare professional charged with the role of safeguarding "looked after" children.

If the embedding of networked technologies in everyday life is an indication of the emergence of the network society (Castells, 2001), then recent findings of the Oxford Internet Institute heralded its arrival in the UK. Internet penetration in the UK has now reached 70% of all households, with 96% of these connections being broadband (Dutton, Helsper, & Gerber, 2009).

Communication is the most commonly cited purpose for Internet use, and the Internet is becoming central to the ways in which people routinely maintain communications with families and friends, locally and at a distance. The authors of the report argue that "the social implications of the Internet are beginning to be increasingly significant, such as in the area of media use and social networking. Perhaps it has begun to approach, if not pass, a tipping point at which the social shaping and implications of the Internet are becoming more apparent" (p. 5).

Among the pioneers of the new networked domain are children and young people, the "digital natives" (Prensky, 2001) who take for granted the opportunities—and risks—associated with constantly connected lifestyles. The Pew Internet American Life project found that 93% of U.S. teenagers between the ages of 12 and 17 were online in 2009 (Lenhart, Purcell, Smith, & Zichuhr, 2010), and the EU (European Union) Kids Online project published evidence of the extensive use of the Internet by children and young people across Europe, including 91% of UK children (Livingstone & Haddon, 2009).

Social networking sites in particular, like MySpace, Bebo, and Facebook, have experienced phenomenal growth. Although much of the recent rapid increase in use has been among adults (Lenhart et al., 2010; Ofcom, 2009), the early settlers were predominantly children and young people who seized the opportunity to occupy a social space that appeared to be under the radar of a risk averse adult society increasingly focused on constraining and controlling their use of physical space (boyd, 2008; Gill, 2008; Valentine, 2004). However, the very affordances that made social networking sites so attractive to young people—allowing online users to communicate and share and exchange text, images, and video with ease—caused growing concern for parents, caregivers, and teachers, whose fears about online pedophiles and cyberbullies were amplified by extreme cases highlighted in the national press (boyd, 2008; Livingstone, 2009; Ponte, Bauwens, & Mascheroni, 2009).

For social workers and others concerned with the welfare of children and young people in the public care system, many of whom are already immersed in a host of offline problems and difficulties as victims and/or perpetrators, the risks of Internet use can seem to outweigh any possible benefits. However, like other aspects of practice in effective social services provision, child care planning should be informed by a careful assessment of the facts of the case and based on evidence of best practice. In the following sections we draw on social science research to describe the nature of the new networked public spaces, the opportunities and risks they present to young people, and the ways in which children and young people are using these spaces. We conclude with a discussion of the particular challenges for social welfare agents cast in the role of "corporate parents."

NETWORKED PUBLIC SPACE

In his article in this special issue, "Social Work and Social Presence in an Online World," LaMendola describes new forms of sociality emerging as part of the rise of the network society. Social networking sites are one manifestation of this phenomenon. In order to clarify the altered nature of communication and community within networked spaces, Ito (2008) and boyd (2008) have referred to the concept of networked publics. Describing online spaces as networked publics emphasizes the communal nature of these spaces and shifts the discourse away from Internet users as passive consumers of media and toward "the ways in which people are networked and mobilized with and through media" (Ito, 2008, p. 2). For boyd (2008), networked publics are both the virtual spaces enabled by networked technologies and "the imagined community that emerges as a result of the intersection of people, technology, and practice" (p. 2). Networked technologies provide affordances for social practices that both extend and alter—sometimes in unexpected ways (e.g., see Houghton & Joinson, "Privacy, Social Network Sites, and Social Relations," in this issue)—the social practices of unmediated public space.

That children and young people have flocked to make use of these networked public spaces is perhaps related to the extent to which—in the developed world—their use of physical public space has become increasingly controlled, managed, and constrained (boyd, 2008; Gill, 2008; Valentine, 2004). For children and young people social networking sites open up new opportunities for relationship building, identity play, informal learning, and creativity (boyd, 2008; Ito et al., 2008; Livingstone, 2009). However, there are concomitant risks associated with these new online spaces. Before exploring the opportunities and risks identified by research we will first describe the characteristics and social dynamics of networked publics.

Based on extensive research into the uses of social networking sites by teenagers, boyd (2008) argues that networked publics have four properties and three dynamics. The properties are characteristics derived from the nature of data capture in digital networks, and the dynamics are related to the social effects of communication in a computer-mediated environment. The four properties of networked publics are: *persistence* (online expressions are automatically recorded and stored over time), *searchability* (content in networked publics can be accessed through search), *replicability* (online content can be copied easily), and *scalability* (the potential visibility of content is global). There are of course technical solutions to constrain the effects of some of these characteristics, such as privacy settings on social networking sites and filters on network access, but it is nonetheless important to note the underlying properties since they provide affordances for many of the opportunities and risks associated with networked publics: these affordances allow communications to be exchanged, shared, and surveilled—now and in the future—in ways that users might not anticipate.

These properties are related to three social dynamics of networked publics described by boyd (2008): *invisible audiences* (not all intended or potential audiences are visible when a person is contributing online), *collapsed contexts* (the lack of spatial, social, and temporal boundaries makes it difficult to maintain distinct social contexts), and the *blurring of public and private* (without control over context, the distinction between public and private becomes problematic).

Issues of privacy, trust, reciprocity, ethics, and intimacy are as central to relationships in networked public spaces as they are face to face, but the technology provides new affordances that can be used for good or ill in equal measure: each opportunity carries a countervailing risk (Livingston, 2009). For example, although participants in a social networking site may have a particular audience in mind when they make contributions, some-times their contributions can be visible to unintended audiences (parents, teachers, social workers, or employers) who may not appreciate the nuanced, contextual nature of the communication. Similarly, sites for the playful construction of identity and the maintenance of trusting, caring relationships can also be used to tease, taunt, bully, and harass (Hinduja & Patchin, 2009).

OPPORTUNITIES AND BENEFITS

Comments in the mass media about young people and social networking sites—often associated with extreme and exceptional cases involving Internet related child abuse or suicide—have helped to fuel a moral panic about the risks associated with these new networked publics (boyd, 2008; Livingstone, 2009; Ponte et al., 2009). Livingstone (2008) captures the situation well when she states, "In short, it is commonly held that at best, social networking is time-wasting and socially isolating and at worst it allows paedophiles to groom children in their bedroom or sees teenagers lured into suicide pacts while parents think they are doing their homework" (p. 395).

In this context it is vitally important that the work of social work and other human service professionals is informed by evidence-based studies of the actual opportunities and risks associated with the Internet and social networking sites. Although there is still much to uncover about this con-stantly evolving phenomenon, a substantial body of evidence has been amassed (e.g., Byron, 2008; Internet Safety Technical Task Force, 2008; Livingstone & Haddon, 2009).

Livingstone and Haddon (2009) analyzed over 400 European research studies on children's use of the Internet. From this data they derived a table describing the opportunities and risks associated with three modes of online communication: *content related* (child as recipient of mass-distributed content), *contact related* (child as participant in an interactive situation predominantly driven by adults), and *conduct related* (child as actor in an interaction in which he or she may be initiator). This classification is particularly helpful in as much as it highlights the young person's role as a creator of opportunities and risks and as a consumer of them. Opportunities included learning and digital literacy, participation and civic engagement, creativity and self-expression, and identity and social connection. Risk areas identified included commercial exploitation, exposure to aggression, risks of a sexual nature, and values based risks (e.g., racist and sexist).

Considering the main risks identified, the authors state that only a very small proportion of teenagers experience an extreme risk, however around 15% to 20% of online teenagers report a degree of distress or a feeling of being uncomfortable or threatened online. Livingstone (2009) summarizes the results of the research pointing out that communicating personal information was quite common and undertaken by about half of all online teenagers. Risks from exposure to content was the next most common risk, especially exposure to sexual or aggressive content (experienced by around 4 in 10 of teenagers across Europe). Contact-related risks varied in incidence with bullying being most common (around 1 in 5 or 6), sexual harassment less common, and meeting online contacts very uncommon (around 9%). Livingstone (2009) recognizes that although the analysis gives some indication of the types of risk and their prevalence it leaves open questions about definition (e.g., of what constitutes pornography), scale (e.g., the extent of distress), interpretation (e.g., whether the experience was unwanted), and benchmarking (i.e., how this compares with pre-Internet risks). The researchers also noted that there were significant gender differences in patterns of exposure to risk:

> Specifically, boys appear more likely to seek out offensive or violent content, to access pornographic content or be sent links to pornographic websites, to meet somebody offline that they have met online and to give out personal information. Girls appear more likely to be upset by offensive, violent and pornographic material, to chat online with strangers, to receive unwanted sexual comments and to be asked for personal information though they are wary of providing it to strangers. Both boys and girls appear at risk of online bullying. (Livingstone & Haddon, 2009, p. 16)

Although this work helps to describe the prevalence of types of risk, Staksrud, Livingstone, Haddon, and Ólafsson (2009) state that it offers an "insufficient understanding of children's own experiences or perspectives...(and) it offers little contextualisation of online activities in children's lives" (p. 3). In the next section we will explore some of the data around the meaning of online activity for children and young people, with a particular focus on the attitudes of young people towards privacy online.

PRIVACY AND INTIMACY IN NETWORKED PUBLICS

One of the most significant misunderstandings adults have of young people's use of networked public space is the widely held view that young people are unconcerned with issues of privacy. The assumption is that if information is made available online then it must be placed there for everyone to see. The research evidence, however, reveals that young people are highly concerned with privacy, but their view of what is important to keep private and from whom may be significantly different from the adult view. To appreciate the differences we need to view young people's activity in the context of their use of social networking sites and recognize that underlying both adult concern and young people's enthusiasm for social networking sites is the relationship between privacy and intimacy. For young people social networking sites provide an opportunity to stay constantly connected with their offline peers, to share experiences, express themselves, and have fun under the radar of an increasingly surveillance-driven adult community. Livingstone (2009) argues that identity is constructed through discourse within intimate relationships, where communication is revealed to intimates and kept private from others.

The teenage bedroom has long been a site where displays of identity, identity play, and the boundaries of privacy and intimacy have been acted out (Lincoln, 2004, 2005, 2006). The media rich, constantly connected, 21st century teenage bedroom—within which 40% of UK 7- to 16-year-olds (Childwise, 2009b) and a third of U.S. teenagers now have Internet-connected computers (Rideout, Foehr, & Roberts, 2010)—is truly a place that "allows teenagers to remove themselves from adult supervision whilst still living with their parents" (Flichy, 1995, p. 165). In addition, the pervasive use of mobile devices—and their ability to connect to social networking sites—means that young people can stay constantly connected wherever they are located. However, the connections that young people are making are focused more on maintaining existing friendship ties than forging links with virtual "friends." The evidence suggests that "youthful practices are best characterised by the flexible intermixing of multiple forms of communication, with online communication primarily used to sustain local friendships already established offline, rather than to make new contacts with distant strangers" (Livingstone & Brake, 2010, p. 76).

Livingstone (2009) argues that revealing some personal information in social networking sites is all part of online identity construction, like keeping a diary, swapping photos, or passing notes in the offline world. Although young people are aware of the possibilities of "stranger danger," their primary privacy concerns appear to be more focused on preventing intrusions into their online space from known adults like parents and teachers (boyd, 2008; Lenhart & Madden, 2007; Livingstone, 2006). In the United States 73% of 12- to 17-year-olds who are online have a social networking profile (Lenhart et al., 2010). In the UK 77% of 7- to 16-year-olds have visited a social networking site, and 59% have their own profile (Childwise, 2009a). Privacy settings are available on most social networking sites, and, partly in response to pressure from child safety advocates, they are growing in sophistication. In the UK 58% of 8- to 17-year-olds make their profile visible to "friends" only (Ofcom, 2008), and in the United States 66% of 12- to 17-year-olds keep their profile partially or wholly private (Lenhart & Madden, 2007). In addition, the U.S. study found that much of the personal information placed in the public domain by young people is either nonrevealing or false. In many cases this misleading information is playful or joking (e.g., claiming to be aged 98), but at the same time it cloaks key aspects of their identity. Although the evidence suggests that young people do make efforts to protect their privacy online, concerns remain about their ability to effectively manage privacy settings on social networking sites (Debatin & Lovejoy, 2009), a problem that could be alleviated by improved site design, offering more contextual help, allowing greater granularity in privacy settings, and making the effects of changes to privacy settings more transparent. A related point here is that it is important for adults not to overstate the actual technical expertise of young people. As the digital domain grows in significance media literacy programs will become increasingly important (O'Neill & Hagen, 2009).

Livingstone (2009) and boyd (2008) argue that young people strive to manage the tension between intimacy and privacy in networked publics. Livingstone suggests that privacy can be defined in different ways: for example, keeping information out of the public domain or determining (controlling or knowing) what information is known to whom. Children and young people she suggests are "most concerned with maintaining their privacy in relation to others within rather than outside their social network" (p. 111). She goes on to suggest, drawing on Takahashi (2008), that the issue from a young person's point of view may be closer to the Japanese opposition between *Uchi* (meaning *inside*, or *us*) and *Soto* (meaning *outside*, or *them*) rather than the Western concept of "public" and "private" where *private* is taken to mean keeping information completely out of the public domain.

In a similar vein Steeves (2009) contrasts Westin's (1967) classic definition of privacy as informational control with a more social definition of privacy that is intimately bound up with human identity and, in the case of children and young people, human development. She draws on Altman's (1975) definition of privacy as an interpersonal event, involving relationships between people, that has three functions or goals: (a) the regulation of interpersonal boundaries, (b) the development and management of interpersonal roles, and (c) self-observation and self-identity.

This social definition of privacy highlights its role in human development and its value for child care professionals. Writing about privacy, in the context of government proposals for a database of all children within the UK, Anderson and colleagues (2007) make the point that privacy is not only a civil right supported in UN (United Nations) Convention on the Rights of the Child but also an essential element in child welfare and child protection:

> Developing a sense of privacy and autonomy in relation to one's personal life is an integral part of becoming a distinct individual. It is thus important that adults maintain a scrupulous respect for privacy in their dealings with children, in order to reinforce personal boundaries and underline each child's right to say "no" to unwanted intrusion. In this way, the right to privacy directly empowers children to protect themselves. (p. 109)

In the final section we explore the challenges of parenting in the network society for corporate parents charged with looking after children and young people in public care. The emphasis will be on the Scottish and UK contexts, but the implications are generalizable to public care elsewhere.

CORPORATE PARENTS AND "LOOKED AFTER" CHILDREN AND YOUNG PEOPLE

Within the UK the term "looked after" is a legal term defining children and young people whose parents are unable to provide ongoing care in either a temporary or a permanent capacity. Children can be looked after as the result of a voluntary agreement between parents and public authorities or as the result of a statutory care order. Children and young people who are looked after may be living with their immediate family, extended family, foster carers, or in residential care. The residential child care sector includes a diverse range of settings from short term-residential units, residential schools, children's homes, and secure units (Elsley, 2008). In 2008 there were over 72.5 thousand looked after children across the UK, with 51.4 thousand in foster care and 10.3 thousand in residential care (The Fostering Network, 2010).

The concept of corporate parenting, first outlined in the Utting Report (Utting, 1997), refers to the state's responsibility for children looked after by local authorities. The language used is a deliberate attempt to encourage state agencies to take their parental responsibilities seriously. The Scottish Government has defined corporate parenting as "the formal and local partnerships needed between all local authority departments and services, and associated agencies, who are responsible for working together to meet the needs of Looked After children and young people, and care leavers" (Scottish Executive, 2007). In England the Department for Education and Skills has stated:

> As the corporate parent of children in the care the State has a special responsibility for their well-being. Like any good parent, it should put its own children first. That means being a powerful advocate for them to receive the best of everything and helping children to make a success of their lives. (Department for Education and Skills, 2006, p. 31)

In the network society successful lives will be media literate lives in which individuals are empowered to make use of Internet for information and advice, use social networking to sustain relationships and build social capital, and be Internet savvy enough to avoid the attendant risks. However, Livingstone (2009) argues that there is a very direct relationship between increasing the opportunities and increasing the risks (Livingstone & Haddon, 2009).

To make matters worse, since many (though not all) young people who are looked after are young people who are at risk offline—young people with low self-esteem, relationship difficulties, and unstable home backgrounds—the evidence suggests they are more likely to be at risk (as victims and/or perpetrators) online. For example, there are indications that children and young people who have low self-esteem or lack satisfying friendships or positive relations with parents may be at higher risk from online social networking (Livingstone & Helsper, 2007; Valkenburg & Peter, 2007; Ybarra & Mitchell, 2004). Young people's use of the Internet and social networking sites does not seem to have led to an increase in sexual predation. Although the context for victimization has changed, the young people at most risk from sexual predation are the same young people at risk from offline harm, including victims of sexual or physical abuse or children from unstable homes (Internet Safety Technical Task Force, 2008). The evidence suggests that cyberstalking by adult offenders, although very concerning, appears to be rare and that most online sexual solicitation of minors derives from other minors and young adults (Internet Safety Technical Task Force, 2008). In relation to the phenomenon of cyberbullying its prevalence appears to be similar to that of offline bullying. Online bullies are around the same age as their victims, and anonymous studies suggest that the majority of perpetrators are known to their victims (Hinduja & Patchin, 2009). However, once again, those children at most risk of involvement in cyberbullying, as victims or perpetrators, are children and young people at risk offline.

This rather depressing—although unsurprising—picture leads Livingstone & Brake (2010) to conclude that "the balance between opportunities and risk should, arguably, be struck differently for "at risk" children, where greater monitoring or restrictions may be legitimate" (p. 6). While it is of great importance to acknowledge the potentially higher risks for looked after children and the greater need for vigilance on the part of corporate parents, it is regrettable that Livingstone and Brake (2010) do not include the need for more intensive supports along with the need for "greater monitoring and restrictions."

The problem is that "greater monitoring or restrictions" sometimes translates into crude technical filtering and monitoring solutions with a blanket ban on social networking sites and network surveillance contracted out to an external IT company with little understanding of the needs of children and young people. Technical solutions have a place but, especially in the absence of other more child-centered strategies, can also provide a false sense of security. They may backfire, particularly with older young people who may enjoy finding ways around crude adult attempts to restrict or monitor Internet usage (Ito et al., 2008).

Instead of relying on technical solutions alone, corporate parents can make use of additional options to enrich their online risk reduction strategies by, for example, (a) running evidence-informed awareness raising campaigns to inform child care staff, foster carers, and young people and opening up discussion about the risks associated with online activities such as cyberbullying (de Haan, 2009); (b) offering programs to improve the media literacy skills of young people and staff (O'Neill & Hagen, 2009); (c) hosting peer-education programs (perhaps involving child advocacy organizations), which may be an effective approach for older and/or more resistant young people (Atkinson, Furnell, & Phippen, 2009); (d) promoting forms of "parental mediation" that combine a blend of technical solutions (involving filtering and monitoring), restrictions, and rule settings (about time, duration, and place of online activity) as well as promoting social approaches (watching, talking, and sharing online activities) linked to age and stage and individual care planning (Kirwil, Garmendia, Garitaonandia, & Fernandez, 2009).

The responsibilities of corporate parents have never been easy. However, whilst recognizing the risks the network society poses for looked-after children and young people, we urge them to consider advice recently issued by the Scottish Government (2008) to corporate parents (which included direct reference to enabling access to social networking sites):

> It is an important part of growing up for children and young people to learn how to take risks, how to take responsibility for themselves and their behaviour and we must be careful not to deny them that opportunity through risk-averse behaviours. Professionals working with children, and particularly senior managers, must strike a balance between protection and preventing young people developing essential life skills. (p. 75)

REFERENCES

Altman, I. (1975). *The environment and social behavior*. Monterey, CA: Brooks/Cole.

Anderson, R., Brown, I., Clayton, R., Dowty, T., Korff, D., & Munro, E. (2007). *Children's Databases—Safety and privacy: A report for the information commissioner*. Wilmslow: Foundation for Information Policy Research.

Atkinson, S., Furnell, S., & Phippen, A. D. (2009, June). *Using peer-education to encourage safe online behaviour. LSE EU Kids Online*. Retrieved from http://www.lse.ac.uk/collections/EUKidsOnline/Conference%20papers.htm

boyd, D. (2008). *Taken out of context: American teen sociality in networked publics*. Doctoral dissertation, University of California, Berkeley.

Byron, T. (2008). *Safer Children in a digital world: the report of the Byron Review*. London: Department for Children, Schools and Families, and the Department for Culture, Media and Sport.

Castells, M. (2001). *The Internet galaxy*. Oxford: Oxford University Press.

ChildWise. (2009a). *The Monitor Report 2008–9: Children's media use and purchasing*. Norwich, UK: ChildWise.

ChildWise. (2009b). *Trends report 2009*. Norwich, UK: ChildWise.

de Hann, J. (2009). Maximising opportunities and minimising risks for children online. In S. Livingstone & L. Haddon (Eds.), *Kids online: Opportunities and risks for children*. Bristol: Policy Press.

Department for Education and Skills. (2006). *Care matters: Transforming the lives of children and young people in care*. Norwich, UK: The Stationery Office.

Debatin, B., & Lovejoy, J. P. (2009). Facebook and online privacy: Attitudes, behaviors, and unintended consequences. *Journal of Computer-Mediated Communication, 15*, 83–108.

Dutton, W. H., Helsper, E. J., & Gerber, M. M. (2009). *Oxford Internet survey 2009 report: The Internet in Britain*. Oxford: Oxford Internet Institute, University of Oxford.

Elsley, S. (2008). *Home truths: Residential child care in Scotland: A context paper*. Glasgow: Scottish Institute for Residential Child Care.

The Fostering Network. (2010). *Foster care statistics 2007–08*. Retrieved from http://www.fostering.net/resources/statistics/foster-care-statistics-2007-08

Flichy, P. (1995). *Dynamics of modern communication: The shaping and impact of new communication technologies*. London: Sage.

Gill, T. (2008). Space-oriented children's policy: Creating child friendly communities to improve children's well-being. *Children and Society, 22*, 136–142.

Hinduja, S., & Patchin, J. (2009). *Bullying beyond the schoolyard: Preventing and responding to cyberbullying*. Thousand Oaks, CA: Corwin Press.

Internet Safety Technical Task Force. (2008). *Enhancing child safety and online technologies: Final report of the internet safety technical task force to the multi-state working group of state attorneys*. Durham, NC: Carolina Academic Press.

Ito, M. (2008). Introduction. In K. Varnelis (Ed.), *Networked publics*. Cambridge, MA: MIT Press.

Ito, M., Horst, H. A., Bittanti, M., Boyd, D., Herr-Stephenson, B., Lange, P. G., et al. (2008). *Living and learning with new media: Summary of findings from the digital youth project*. The John D. and Catherine T. MacArthur Foundation Reports on Digital Media and Learning. Retrieved from http://digitalyouth. ischool.berkeley.edu/report

Kirwil, L., Garmendia, M., Garitaonandia, C., & Fernandez, G. M. (2009). Parental mediation. In S. Livingstone & L. Haddon (Eds.), *Kids online: Opportunities and risks for children*. Bristol: Policy Press.

Lenhart, A., & Madden, M. (2007). Teens, privacy, and online social networkings: How teens manage their online identities and personal information in the age of MySpace. Pew Internet and American Life Project. Retrieved from http://www. pewInternet.org/Reports/2007/Teens-Privacy-and-Online-Social-Networks.aspx

Lenhart, A., Purcell, K., Smith, A., & Zichuhr, K. (2010). Social media and mobile Internet use among teens and young adults. *Pew Internet and American Life Project*. Retrieved from http://www.pewInternet.org/Reports/2010/ Social-Media-and-Young-Adults.aspx

Lincoln, S. (2004). Teenage girl's bedroom culture: Codes versus zones. In A. Bennett & K. Harris (Eds.), *Beyond subculture: Critical commentaries on subcultural theory*. Hampshire: Palgrave.

Lincoln, S. (2005). Feeling the noise: Teenagers, bedrooms and music. *Leisure Studies, 24*(4), 399–414.

Lincoln, S. (2006). Beyond bedrooms?. In T. Palmaarts (Ed.), *Talkie walkie: Jonger-ensubcultuur believers/non-believers*. Leuven: Acco Publishers.

Livingstone, S. (2006). Children's privacy online. In R. Kraut, M. Brynin, & S. Kiesler (Eds.), *Computers, phones, and the Internet: Domesticating information technologies*. New York: Oxford University Press.

Livingstone, S. (2008). Taking risky opportunities in youthful content creation: Teenagers' use of social networking sites for intimacy, privacy and self-expression. *New Media & Society, 10*(3), 393–411.

Livingstone, S. (2009). *Children and the Internet*. Cambridge: Polity Press.

Livingstone, S., & Brake, D. R. (2010). On the rapid rise of social networking sites: New findings and policy implications. *Children and Society, 24*(1), 75–83.

Livingstone, S., & Haddon, L. (2009). *EU kids online: Final report*. London: EU Kids Online.

Livingstone, S., & Helsper, E. J. (2007). Taking risks when communicating on the Internet: The role of offline social-psychological factors in young people's vulnerability to online risks. *Information, Communication and Society, 10*(5), 619–643.

Ofcom. (2008). *Social networking: A quantitative and qualitative report into attitudes, behaviours and use*. London: Office of Communications. Retrieved from http://www.ofcom.org.uk/advice/media_literacy/medlitpub/medlitpubrss/ socialnetworking/

Ofcom. (2009). *UK adults' media literacy: Interim report*. Londong: Office of Communications. Retrieved from http://www.ofcom.org.uk/advice/media_literacy/ medlitpub/medlitpubrss/uk_adults_ml/

O'Neill, B., & Hagen, I. (2009). Media literacy. In S. Livingstone & L. Haddon (Eds.), *Kids online: Opportunities and risks for children*. Bristol: Policy Press.

Ponte, C., Bauwens, J., & Mascheroni, G. (2009). Children and the Internet in the news: Agency, voices and agendas. In S. Livingstone & L. Haddon (Eds.), *Kids online: Opportunities and risks for children*. Bristol: Policy Press.

Prensky, M. (2001). Digital natives, digital immigrants. *On the Horizon, 9*(5), 1–10.

Rideout, V. J., Foehr, U. G., & Roberts, D. F. (2010). *Generation M2: Media in the lives of 8 to 18 year olds.* Menlo Park, CA: Kaiser Family Foundation.

The Scottish Government. (2008). *These are our Bairns: A guide for community planning partnerships on being a good corporate parent.* Edinburgh: Author.

Scottish Executive. (2007). *Looked after children and young people: We can and must do better.* Edinburgh: Author.

Staksrud, E., Livingstone, S., Haddon, L., & Ólafsson, K. (2009). *What do we know about children's use of online technologies? A report on data availability and research gaps in Europe,* (2nd ed.). London: EU Kids Online.

Steeves, V. (2009). Reclaiming the social value of privacy. In I. Kerr, V. Steeves & C. L. Kerr (Eds.), *Lessons from the identity trail: Anonymity, privacy and identity in a networked society.* Oxford: Oxford University Press.

Takahashi, T. (2008). *Japanese young people, media, and everyday life: Towards the de Westernising of media studies.* In K. Drotner & S. Livingstone (Eds.), *International Handbook of Children, Media and Culture.* London: Sage.

Utting, Sir, W. (1997). *People like us—The report of the review of the safeguards for children living away from home.* London: Department of Health.

Valentine, G. (2004). *Public space and the culture of childhood.* Hants, UK: Ashgate.

Valkenburg, P. M., & Peter, J. (2007). Internet communication and its relationship to well-being: Identifying some underlying mechanisms. *Media Psychology, 9*(1), 43–58.

Westin, A. (1967). *Privacy and freedom.* New York: Atheneum.

Ybarra, M. L., & Mitchell, K. J. (2004). Online aggressor/targets, aggressors, and targets: A comparison of associated youth characteristics. *Journal of Child Psychology and Psychiatry, 45*(7), 1308.

Social Work and Social Presence in an Online World

WALTER LAMENDOLA

University of Denver, Denver, Colorado

Human presence is a fundamental consideration of social work practices. The argument in this article is not to undermine such notions but to elaborate on them based on research into social presence, a type of presence projected when a person is associating with others. Communication and information technologies support applications that develop social presence and enable sociality. Such forms of presence are not confined to face-to-face encounters but are necessarily relational. Underlying such a realization is the conviction that all flows of social presence must and can be connected and directed in the conduct of social work practices.

INTRODUCTION

In the United States, the traditional view is that social work grew through two European roots in the mid-1800s: the Charity Organization Societies and the settlement movement. Shortly thereafter, by the end of the 19th century, social work classes were being taught at Columbia University in New York City. Roy Lubove (1965) was one of a number of historians who argued that social work developed in the United States as volunteers working in charitable roles became scarce. Lubove believed that the pressures of modernity contributed to the formation of both the occupation and "agencies," formal organizations who acted as agents for the needy. For him, the origins of social work were moralistic and personal, but its movement forward was bureaucratic, with "casework" increasingly emphasized as a hallmark feature of the profession. Seth Koven and Sonja Michel (1990) argue otherwise, pointing out that the emergence of social welfare programs and policies coincided with the rise of maternalism and the success of women's social action movements. Indeed, a number of women, such as Jane Addams, emerged in the United States and Europe who had the vision as well as the political and financial resources to successfully promote social welfare and social policies. But it is the case that regardless of their impetus, new social welfare policies and practices produced new forms of social relationships in the United States, most notably between the law and women and children, between the immigrant and their new neighbors, and between the school and family.

New social welfare policies were assembled and carried out by some old professions, like nursing and teaching, but also by an emerging one, social work. In effect, social workers, with their focus on face-to-face visits, signified a new *presence* of the modern world in the lives of the poor, the immigrant, the worker, the farmer, the sick, and children. This type of work involved an ethic in visitation that was gradually disconnected from any moralistic judgment though not from intent, comparable if not similar to what Levinas (1969) called *the experience of the encounter*. For our purposes here, it is enough to say that Levinas explains *the experience of the encounter* as a privileged face-to-face phenomenon in which those involved realize their ethical responsibilities to one another. Levinas argues further that *presence*—physical presence felt as both closeness and separation—is important in our encounters with others. For Levinas, the encounter demanded physical presence. Certainly physical presence is important. Riva, Waterworth, and Waterworth (2004) describe it as a defining feature of self and relate the sense of presence to the evolution of a key feature of any central nervous system: the embedding of sensory-referred properties into an internal functional space. They argue that without the emergence of the sense of presence it is impossible for the nervous system to identify the separation between an external world and the internal one. Therefore the notion of Levinas is important for many reasons, only one of which is that it speaks to human presence as a fundamental consideration of social work practices. For social work as for Levinas, human presence conveys a relationship of caring and responsibility for the other in ethical patterns of involvement and aspiration for human realization. The argument in this paper is not to undermine or subvert such a notion of the sense of presence but to elaborate it. In this elaboration I confine myself to only one "strata" or layer of the form of presence known as *social presence*, a type of presence projected when a person is associating with others. Social presence has been the subject of extensive research that is discussed more fully later in the paper. Such a form of presence is not confined to face-to-face encounters but is necessarily relational, motivated by individual aspiration and directed toward involvement with others.

HUMAN NETWORKS

Patterns of relational involvement and human aspiration are a central concern of social work. Bruno LaTour (2005) has written about human patterns of involvement in a manner that fits well with the practice of social work. He points out that the word *social* refers not only to the already constructed forms of association that humans have created, such as families, communities, or organizations, but also to the process of assembling or reassembling human association(s) into different forms. Social work is active in both senses of the word. Social workers associate others in individual ways (finding a child who is neglected and providing a safe place for them) and in ways that influence communities (they help form a neighborhood group to support immigrant families) and organizations (they form an nongovernmental organization or nonprofit to provide services to the homeless). Though it is not all that they do, much of what social workers have done traditionally involves associating and reassembling social relations or creating new ones. LaTour (2005) has argued that such activities have been neglected as a topic of social science and calls for a *sociology of associations* that focuses on human networks (p. 9).

It is certainly true that on a larger scale, such as those that represent LaTour's human network interests, the nature, quality, and type of association that are available to us in the Western world have multiplied in the past few generations and are the subject of considerable interest. Of course, in the title of this article I refer to only a portion of the possibilities when I use the term "online." More expansive possibilities were noted by observers like Van Dijk (2006) who claimed that what he called the "network society" was one in which face-to-face communication would be supplemented and sometimes replaced by associations developed through digital forms of communication. A few years later, Castells (1996) in the first book of a trilogy titled *The Information Age: Economy, Society, and Culture* noted that there was something radically different between associations made in older forms of human networks and those appearing through the personal use of locally situated and widely distributed electronic devices. The radical difference led him to the conclusion that those networks would soon become the fundamental organizing points of society, not the individual, family, organizations, or the state.

In the United States, among the most generative early examples of technology supported human networks were those of Hiltz and Turoff (1978) at the New Jersey Institute of Technology. Hiltz and Turoff were among an early group of innovators who recognized that with nothing more than linked computer mediated communications, participants reported the experience of a *sense of community*. For example, social workers involved in the first invited conference on information technology in social work at

Wingspread (Geiss & Viswanathan, 1985) used Turoff's New Jersey Electronic Information Exchange System (EIES). Though it may have been unusual for the time, they planned, coordinated, and carried out the conference with only a few face-to-face and many asynchronous communication sessions. EIES was perhaps primitive by today's standards, but the outcome of EIES use was an effective community building experience for those involved (Hiltz, 1994).

SOCIAL PRESENCE

While Turoff, Hilz, and others studied the development of communities of different kinds using computer mediated communications, earlier empirical work by social psychologists John Short, Ederyn Williams, and Bruce Christie (1976) had investigated their theory that communication could convey an "awareness" of the other person. They called the awareness they noted *social presence*. They defined social presence as a property of the medium that indicated "the degree of salience of the other person in a mediated communication and the consequent salience of their interpersonal interactions" (p. 76). Their initial investigation has spawned more than 40 years of research and redefinition, as the construct of social presence seems deeper, stratified, and more comprehensive than the original research envisioned. For example, researchers have noted that social presence might include your perceptions of the degree to which you feel you are (a) being there, with others, together; (b) being involved and known; and/or (c) being immediately engaged in activities (Biocca, Harms, & Burgoon, 2003). The overview of Biocca, Harms, and Burgoon illuminates the variability of past research that attempts to deal with both the mediation of the computer networks, as well as of the behavior of those who participate in such interactions.

Ruth Rettie, in a series of published works over the past six years, has taken a slightly different path in denoting three meanings of *social presence*. These three meanings are of special interest to social work, particularly since one point of departure is Goffman's notion of presence as limited to face-to-face interaction (Rettie, 2005). Rettie's three meanings include the use of social presence to refer to the projected presence of a person. The second use of the term that she defines refers to the *experience* of being present. The third use of the term is as *copresence*, referring to the psychological connection that is established when users feel that they have access to the other person's affect and intentions and believe that the other person is "there" (p. 2).

In the first sense a person makes their presence known through a series of activities that relate to the technologies that they are using; for example, they dial a telephone number, and when it is answered they sense the presence of others. In the second use of the term, the experience happens as, in the example of telephone use, social interactions take place—the telephone conversation. In the third sense of the term, Rettie suggests that we distinguish *copresence* as the "mutual awareness of each other by the participants in an interaction" (p. 3). An example may be the affect and cues that people give one another about their feelings and intentions during a telephone conversation. Rettie (2009) goes on to argue that

> a phone call affords a degree of mutual monitoring, warrants focused attention.... There appear to be two different types of mediated contact: communication such as mail, which may occur incidentally within an existing situation but which does not create an intersubjective social experience, and communication such as a phone call, which is more similar to a face-to-face encounter. Synchronous continuous media, such as phone calls and video links, enable a degree of ongoing mutual monitoring in real-time. Although the interactants are in different locations, they share a time-frame and a mediated copresence: as the interactants converse they collaborate on what we can call a *mediated encounter*. (emphasis mine) (p. 425)

This brief introduction to Rettie's notion of social presence betrays the complexity that is the subject of her current research. But for our purposes, the introduction is taken as sufficient to argue the importance of the concept to social work. It elaborates social presence in such a manner that one can extend the ethic of the encounter and *copresence* from face-to-face encounters to *mediated encounters*.

One manner of detailing such an elaboration of social presence is to examine the discursive cues that present themselves in mediated communications. This has seemed a fundamental consideration, particularly since Short, Williams, and Christie (1976) described social presence as a *constellation of cues* (p. 157). Garrison and Anderson (2003) later constructed a classification scheme that describes three broad categories of social presence cues in a mediated conversation:

- Affective responses, such as expressions of emotions, use of humor, and self disclosure
- Open communication responses, such as asking questions, expressing agreement, and complimenting others
- Cohesive responses, such as referring to others by name, addressing the group as "we," and personal greetings (p. 33)

For example, one could speculate that social work service users who perceive an online discussion to be lacking social presence in terms of the cues as proposed would likely not choose the group for engagement. The argument might be that participants in an online conversation, for example, would judge whether their *voice* is heard by others, how "open" the others were, and whether the conversation "was going anywhere."

In sum, I think that the approach to social presence I am developing here has at least five elements of interest to social work, if not all human services. First, it positions social presence as foundational to extracting a sense of the other people involved in the communication and in making decisions that relate to establishing and trusting the relationship. Second, it implies that social presence contributes to the determination of the nature and type of relationship that will be maintained. Third, from a practical perspective it is, in and of itself, a "triggering event" to the extent that subjective judgment and reflection is applied to each communication (Garrison, 2007). Fourth, it awards a formative role to social presence that influences future communications and future subjective judgments. Fifth, social presence seems critical to the formation of community (Gunawardena & Zittle, 1997; Richardson & Swan, 2003; Rovai, 2002).

It is perhaps the following point that has surprising interest to social work: the commonplace recognition that the online world is, in part, a world of social networks that promote community. As Wellman (2001) argued:

> Computer networks are inherently social networks, linking people, organizations, and knowledge. They are social institutions that should not be studied in isolation but as integrated into everyday lives. The proliferation of computer networks has facilitated a deemphasis on group solidarities at work and in the community and afforded a turn to networked societies that are loosely bounded and sparsely knit. The Internet increases people's social capital, increasing contact with friends and relatives who live nearby and far away. New tools must be developed to help people navigate and find knowledge in complex, fragmented, networked societies. (p. 2031)

If one accepts Wellman's argument, "computer networks" (social networks) had become "social institutions" integrated into "everyday lives" and as such emerged as an important concern of social work practice no later than the turn of the 21st century. In fact, McNutt (2000) pointed out social work practice concerns that dealt with computer networking at about that time. But also note well that Wellman claims network societies of the time to be "sparsely knit." Furthermore, as a social worker I take his conclusion as a charge to social work, much like that taken up by the settlement houses: to develop "new tools" to "help people navigate and find knowledge" in the birthing of a new culture propelled by mediated encounters.

LIQUEFYING DISTANCE

To continue the argument of a charge being laid at the foot of the social work discipline, I take the context of the charge to be that social work needs to confront the changes in culture that are taking place. As in the settlement house era though larger in scale, inequities, oppression, mass migrations, and displacements are taking place. There are, it seems, many reasons why social work would need to take notice. A fundamental perception of the drivers of current cultural changes has been articulated as ones that involve mobility. This notion has been explored for over two decades now (Urry & Lash, 1987; Urry, 2007). The approach views culture as developing in a world of flows rather than places. For example, these could be *social flows* of people, information, ideas, video, and images. Social scientists would contend that evidence of cultural development is seen through forms of social formation (Archer, 1996). For example, Facebook participation can mobilize "flows" of friendships and communities, and social formation demands human encounters of all types.

Earlier in this article I described the human encounter as one of caring and responsibility for the other. In its maturity, participants gather in ethical patterns of involvement and aspiration for human realization. Encounters that take place in a condition of cultural infancy may be a different story (Lanier, 2010). Lanier makes what could be called a developmental cultural argument when he calls our present experience of mediated encounters one of "wave after wave of juvenilia" (p. 182). He goes on to argue that nothing is particularly wrong or unexpected with our cultural infancy but that it is infancy and that it does with a "dark side" of crime, bullying, and general mayhem. Kreijns, Kirschner, and Jochems (2003) had made similar arguments earlier, observing that designers of software used in mediated encounters had taken for granted ethical and psychological considerations in the belief that people should socially interact simply because the environment makes it possible. They identified a tendency by software developers to restrict social formation assisted by software in a manner that ignored emotional and contextual considerations. By doing so, software developers created mediated environments that neglected *social* dimensions of the desired social interaction, such as how interpersonal communication is altered by the software; how social interactions contribute to group development; how group cohesion, trust, respect, and belonging are critical elements of the emerging social space; and how a sense of community and the ensuing social capital must be managed. They end their article by pointing out that considerations of social presence in mediated encounters are more important than the same considerations in face-to-face-environments (p. 336).

Even further, the latest analysis by Castells (2009) depicts the network society as exclusionary, where those involved in mediated networks are living a space of *flows*, whereas those who are uninvolved live in a space of *places* (p. 50). Harry Ferguson (2008) pointed out that mobilities and flows were an important consideration for social work. In a prescient article on liquid social work, he argued that social workers "need to understand much more about how the diverse mobilities of social work and welfare practices shape the patterning of professional work and service users' lives and influence the effectiveness of what is done, creating opportunities and dangers" (p. 563). While Ferguson errs by limiting the flow and mobility involved in the conduct of social work to physical movement, his diagnosis is sound. The point is that social work increasingly involves mobile, emerging encounters, but in both place and space (Urry, 2000). Encounters are not limited to Ferguson's examples of a car or office; they are increasingly characterized by different forms of presence, such as cell phones, YouTube, Facebook, and other software applications (Wellman & Haythornthwaite, 2002). In LaTour's (2005) metaphorical terms, these forms of presence carry the subject and people flow from individual action to attachments. For example, imagine the cell phone as a portable community. The flow of cell phone use can be quite complex in any given day. For example, at any moment a social worker can be talking to a service user, to members of a troubled family, texting colleagues, participating in case conference video calls, or commenting with other agency staff on an Internet posting. Clearly, social workers must come to understand that a part of working with the social in a network society is to be:

- inherently connected with mobile encounters involving communication and surveillance, which form complex flows of presence and absence;
- involved with portable communities where sociality flows in and out of space or fills and empties space creating conversational buckets, streams of intimacy, and narrative torrents; and
- a geographer of the ebb and flow of human potentials and perversities across a torrent of networked social practices.

THE SCIENCE OF ASSOCIATION

Up to this point, I have laid out what I consider to be important elements of an argument that of all the human services, social work is distinguished by engaging in what LaTour (2005) called the *science of associations*. Ferguson correctly notes the associative base of social work and the value of face-to-face communication such as home visiting and then limits copresence to physical presence. This would be a mistake. I think it is time to expand our understanding and use of presence. And though social workers have just begun their explorations of the practical use and application of forms of presence, the expanded capacity to manipulate presence in working with the social is possibly the most important contribution of convergent technologies to social work so far.

Many of the social work challenges for new practice development lie in the examination of the manner in which people form associations in a network society, particularly in mediated encounters. In this regard, one of the most important concepts underlying such an approach is sociality. *Sociality* is a term that originates in the biological sciences and has more recently found wider use in the design of "social" software that "allows for social relations in cyberspace that are nearly as rich and meaningful as those in real life" (Bouman et al., 2008). Social scientists dating back to Meade (1938) have variously defined *sociality* as an activity whereby human actors relate to one another to form groups, organize social practices, and construct their identities (Krause & Ruxton, 2002). If one were to accept the argument that sociality is an activity of developing associations, then perhaps the place to look for new tools to work with people will come from studying those interactions (Kaptelinin & Nardi, 2006). In this regard, one could consider social presence as an activity that is conducted in the service of achieving sociality, and there can be no doubt that those activities can and do take place in the "online world." They are so common that one could hypothesize that sociality is one of the primary human purposes of participation in a network society.

Of course, such a claim is not unique. We now uniformly call Web 2.0 software "social" software and the present form of the Web the *social Web* (Boulos & Wheelert, 2007). Boulos and Wheelert review available software applications that characterize social software based on activities that indicate human presence. Some of these activities have emerging practices by which humans perform sociality critical to social work, such as:

- participation and inquiry,
- identity and affiliation
- primary and private relationships, and
- association and social action.

SUMMARY

In many cases the issues and challenges of emerging social work practice in a network society are human issues in all societies and already known to social work, such as ethics, trust, responsibility, reciprocation, obligation, isolation, common good, common interest, reciprocity, participation, and evil. Petrovcic (2008) enumerates a number of studies in regard to these, studies that indicate that active participation online leads to larger personal networks for emotional support, that proximity is still an important resource for emotional and physical support, that higher mobile phone use equals more visits to relatives, and that more active users tend to have higher voluntary organization participation. Across any number of personal networks, practices emerge with use and human activity with computing artifacts commonly results in unanticipated practices. New forms of sociality emerge facilitated by the practices people develop when they play and experiment with different forms of technology mediation.

In an online world, social presence symbolizes the imprint of humanity and the embodied need for our kind to associate. It is not a sign of human abandonment. Castells (2009) traces the vein of human engagement when he says that:

> citizens of the Information Age become able to invent new programs for their lives with the materials of their suffering, fears, dreams, and hopes. They build their projects by sharing their experience. They subvert the practice of communication as usual by squatting in the medium and creating their message. They overcome the powerlessness of their solitary despair by networking their desire. They fight the powers that be by identifying the networks that are . . . if you think differently, communication networks will operate differently. (pp. 431–432)

For social work to begin to move forward, the discipline's work with the social must engage intimately with the practices of everyday life, with where life flows. Social work has a need to establish firm footing in all spaces where humans create associations, whether online or off line. But an expanded notion of presence for the profession means blending face-to-face encounters with those that are not. It means accepting the premise that social presence is embodied but not contained by physicality. It is an appreciation that in all its forms, social presence is the carrier of relationships. Forms of social presence are powerful human tools that provide a basis for sociality, such as our need to relate, to associate with others. In this article I have dealt only with raising our collective social work consciousness about forms of social presence that support sociality by relying on communication and information technology mediation. However, underlying such a position is the conviction that all flows of social presence must and can be connected and directed in the conduct of social work practice.

REFERENCES

Archer, M. (1996). *Culture and agency*, (Revised ed.). New York: Cambridge University Press.

Biocca, F., Harms, C., & Burgoon, J. (2003). Toward a more robust theory and measure of social presence: Review and suggested criteria. *Presence*, *12*(5), 456–480.

Boulos, M. N. K., & Wheelert, S. (2007). The emerging Web 2.0 social software: An enabling suite of sociable technologies in health and healthcare education. *Health Information and Libraries Journal*, *24*(1), 2–23.

Bouman, W., Hoogenboom, T., Jansen, R., Schoondorp, M., de Bruin, B., & Huizing, A. (2008). "The realm of sociality: Notes on the design of social software," University of Amsterdam, Netherlands. *Sprouts: Working Papers on Information Systems*, *8*(1). Retrieved from http://sprouts.aisnet.prg/8–1

Castells, M. (1996). *The Information Age: Economy, society and culture* (vol. I)*: The rise of the network society*. Oxford: Blackwell.

Castells, M. (2009). *Communication power.* New York: Oxford University Press.

Ferguson, H. (2008). Liquid social work: Welfare interventions as mobile practices. *British Journal of Social Work, 38*, 561–579.

Garrison, D. R. (2007). Online community of inquiry review: Social, cognitive, and teaching presence issues. *Journal of Asynchronous Learning Networks, 11*(1), 61–72.

Garrison, D. R., & Anderson, T. (2003). *E-learning in the 21st century: A framework for research and practice.* New York: Routledge Falmer.

Geiss, G., & Viswanathan, N. (Eds.) (1985). *The human edge: Information technology and helping people.* Binghamton, NY: The Haworth Press.

Gunawardena, C. N., & Zittle, F. J. (1997). Social presence as a predictor of satisfaction within computer mediated conferencing environment. *American Journal of Distance Education, 11*(3), 8–26.

Hiltz, S. R. (1994). *The virtual classroom: Learning without limits using the virtual classroom.* Norwood, NJ: Ablex Pub. Corp.

Hiltz, S. R., & Turoff, M. (1978). *The network nation.* Reading, MA: Addison-Wesley.

Kaptelinin, V., & Nardi, B. (2006). *Acting with technology: Activity theory and interaction design.* London: MIT Press.

Koven, S., & Michel, S. (1990). Womanly duties: Maternalist politics and the origins of welfare states in France, Germany, Great Britain, and the United States, 1880–1920. *The American Historical Review, 95*(4), 1076–1108.

Krause, J., & Ruxton, G. D. (2002). *Living in groups.* New York: Oxford University Press.

Kreijns, K., Kirschner, P. A., & Jochems, W. (2003). Identifying the pitfalls for social interaction in computer-supported collaborative learning environments: A review of the research. *Computers in Human Behavior, 19*, 335–353.

Lanier, J. (2010). *You are not a gadget.* New York: Knopf.

LaTour, B. (2005). *Reassembling the social: An introduction to actor network theory.* New York: Oxford University Press.

Levinas, E. (1969). *Totality and infinity: An essay on exteriority.* (A. Lingis, Trans.). Pittsburgh: Duquesne University Press. (Original work published 1961.)

Lubove, R. (1965). *The professional altruist.* Cambridge: Harvard University Press.

McNutt, J. (2000). Organizing cyberspace: Strategies for teaching about community practice and technology. *Journal of Community Practice, 7*(1), 95–109.

Meade, G. (1938). *The philosophy of the act.* (C.W. Morris, Ed.) Chicago: University of Chicago Press.

Petrovcic, A. (2008). Reconfiguring socialities: The personal networks of ICT users and social cohesion. *tripleC, 6*(2), 146–166.

Rettie, R. (2005). Social presence as presentation of self (sketch 16, working paper 17). 8th Annual International Workshop on Presence, London, September 21–23.

Rettie, R. (2009). Mobile phone communication: Extending Goffman to mediated interaction. *Sociology, 43*, 421–438.

Richardson, J., & Swan, K. (2003). Examining social presence in online courses in relation to students' perceived learning and satisfaction. *Journal of Asynchronous Learning Network, 7*(1), 68–88.

Riva, G., Waterworth, J. A., & Waterworth, E. L. (2004). The layers of presence: A bio-cultural approach to understanding presence in natural and mediated environments. *CyberPsychology & Behavior, 7*(4), 402–416.

Rovai, A. P. (2002). Sense of community, perceived cognitive learning, and persistence in asynchronous learning networks. *The Internet and Higher Education, 5*(4), 319–332.

Short, J., Williams, E., & Christie, B. (1976). *The social psychology of telecommunications.* London: John Wiley & Sons.

Urry, J. (2000). *Sociology beyond societies: Mobilities for the twenty-first century.* New York: Routledge.

Urry, J. (2007). *Mobilities.* Cambridge: Polity.

Urry, J., & Lash, S. (1987). *The end of organized capitalism.* Madison, WI: University of Wisconsin Press.

Van Dijk, J. A. G. M. (2006). *The network society: Social aspects of the new media* (2nd ed.). London: Sage. (Original Dutch edition 1991.)

Wellman, B. (2001). Computer networks as social networks. *Science, 293,* 2031–2034.

Wellman, B., & Haythornthwaite, C. (Eds.) (2002). *The Internet in everyday life. Malden,* MA: Blackwell Publishing.

Index

Page numbers in *Italics* represent tables.

INDEX

top-down model 19–21; ATM 19; concerted suboptimization 20; description 19–20; global banking infrastructure 19–21; impact on practice 20; information-sharing infrastructure 19–20; social workers 20, 24
travel websites 18
Tunstall 49, 57
Turoff, M. 114; and Hiltz, S.R. 113–14

Uncertainty Reduction Theory (URT) 86–7
United Kingdom (UK): Internet 98; young people and SNS 104
United Nations (UN) 7
United States of America (USA): IGHI 13–14; society 6; total information awareness 42; young people and SNS 104

Van Dijk, J.A.G.M. 1, 114
Virilio, P. 28, 38–9, 41

Warren, S.V.: and Brandeis, L.D. 87

Waterworth, E.L.: Riva, G. and Waterworth, J.A. 112
Webb, L.T.: *et al* 4
Wellman, B. 2, 116
Westin, A.F. 79, 89
Wheelert, S.: and Boulos, M.N.K. 119
Whitaker, R. 42
Whole-System Demonstrator Programme 73
Williams, E.: Christie, B. and Short, J. 114, 115
Wilmot, S. 52
Winkler, M. 40

York Health Economics Consortium (YHEC) 65
young people: care system 99; internet usage 99, 101–2
young people and SNS 101–3, 106; activity 103; enthusiasm 103; identity 103; mobile devices 103; online risk reduction strategies 107; opportunities 102; privacy 103–4; risks 101–2, 106–7; role 102; UK 104; USA 104

Printed and bound by CPI Group (UK) Ltd, Croydon, CR0 4YY

21/10/2024

01777040-0005